Carcinoma of the Breast

Edited by

Carl J. D'Orsi, M.D.
Professor and Vice Chairman,
Department of Radiology,
University of Massachusetts Medical School;
Radiologist, University of Massachusetts
Medical Center, Worcester

Richard E. Wilson, M.D.
Professor of Surgery,
Harvard Medical School;
Chief, Surgical Oncology,
Brigham and Women's Hospital and
Sidney Farber Cancer Institute,
Boston

Carcinoma of the Breast: Diagnosis and Treatment

Little, Brown and Company
Boston / Toronto

Contents

Contributing Authors

Nelson A. Burstein, M.D.
Associate Professor of Pathology, Tufts University School of Medicine; Director of Laboratories, St. Elizabeth's Hospital, Boston

George P. Canellos, M.D.
Professor of Medicine, Harvard Medical School; Chief, Medical Oncology, Sidney Farber Cancer Institute, Boston

Carl J. D'Orsi, M.D.
Professor and Vice Chairman, Department of Radiology, University of Massachusetts Medical School; Radiologist, University of Massachusetts Medical Center, Worcester

Christopher C. Gates, M.D.
Staff Psychiatrist, New England Deaconess Hospital, Boston

Jay R. Harris, M.D.
Associate Professor of Radiation Therapy, Harvard Medical School; Clinical Director, Joint Center for Radiation Therapy, Boston

Samuel Hellman, M.D.
Professor and Chairman, Department of Radiation Therapy, Harvard Medical School; Director, Joint Center for Radiation Therapy, Boston

I. Craig Henderson, M.D.
Assistant Professor of Medicine, Harvard Medical School; Medical Coordinator, Breast Evaluation Center, Sidney Farber Cancer Institute, Boston

William D. Kaplan, M.D.
Associate Professor of Radiology, Harvard Medical School; Chief, Oncologic Nuclear Medicine, Sidney Farber Cancer Institute, Boston

Jennifer L. Kelsey, Ph.D.
Associate Professor of Epidemiology and Public Health, Yale University School of Medicine, New Haven, Connecticut

†Martin B. Levene, M.D.
Formerly Associate Professor of Radiation Therapy, Harvard Medical School; Deputy Director, Joint Center for Radiation Therapy, Boston

†Deceased

Robert T. Osteen, M.D.
> *Assistant Professor of Surgery, Harvard Medical School; Junior Associate in Surgery, Brigham and Women's Hospital, Boston*

Edward H. Smith, M.D.
> *Professor and Chairman, Department of Radiology, University of Massachusetts Medical School; Radiologist, University of Massachusetts Medical Center, Worcester*

Aziza Soliman-Fam, M.D., Ph.D.
> *Associate Professor of Anatomy, Harvard Medical School, Boston*

Richard E. Wilson, M.D.
> *Professor of Surgery, Harvard Medical School; Chief, Surgical Oncology, Brigham and Women's Hospital and Sidney Farber Cancer Institute, Boston*

Preface

This book attempts to present the many facets of breast carcinoma diagnosis and treatment in a single, readable source. While several books deal separately and exhaustively with the various topics included here, there is also a real need for one book designed to present all of the topics in some detail and to stimulate further reading as necessary.

The contributors to this volume are all recognized authorities in their respective fields. The chapter on psychological aspects of breast cancer by Christopher Gates and the chapter on biochemical markers by Nelson Burstein are unique in a book on breast cancer.

It is our hope that this book will provide a complete overview of breast carcinoma for the senior medical student, intern, and resident, all of whom most certainly will deal with this disease during their careers.

C. J. D.
R. E. W.

Carcinoma of the Breast

Jennifer L. Kelsey

1. Epidemiology of Breast Cancer in Women

Breast cancer is a major public health problem for women in the United States and other Western countries. In the United States, the annual age-adjusted incidence rate is about 85 per 100,000 women, and the age-adjusted mortality is about 28 per 100,000 women [154]; each year more than 100,000 women are diagnosed as having breast cancer, and about 30,000 deaths are attributable to it. It has been estimated [187] that 1 in every 14 women in the United States will develop breast cancer at some time during her life. Although mortality has remained relatively constant for many years, incidence rates have been increasing over the past two decades [10, 45].

Demographic Characteristics of Cases

In the United States and other Western industrialized countries, incidence rates for breast cancer increase rapidly with age until about 45 to 50 years of age; after this they continue to increase but at a slower rate [57]. Whites are affected somewhat more frequently than blacks [184]; Jews are affected more frequently than non-Jews [144, 184]; and women in upper social classes are affected more frequently than women in lower social classes [41, 55]. Women who have never been married are at greater risk than women who have been married, and nulliparous women are at higher risk than women who have borne children [95, 110, 144]. Within the United States, women living in urban areas are more likely to develop breast cancer than those in rural localities, and rates are higher in the North than in the South [22].

About 1 percent of breast cancer cases have simultaneous primary tumors in both breasts [23]. Unilateral tumors occur more frequently in the left breast than in the right breast, with the ratio of tumors in the left breast to the right ranging from 1.05 to 1.20 in various studies [62, 115]. Although the excess on the left side has been reported in many countries and in different racial groups, the reason for this excess is not known.

1

International Variation

In general, low incidence rates and mortality for breast cancer have been reported in most Asian and African countries, while intermediate rates have been found in southern European and South American countries, and high rates occur in North American and northern European countries [52]. It is of further interest that in most North American and northern European countries, incidence rates for breast cancer increase over the entire age span, with a somewhat less rapid rate of increase with age after 45 to 54 years of age than before (see Fig. 1–1). In countries with intermediate incidence rates and mortality, the incidence rates tend to plateau after about 50 years of age. In countries in which the risk for breast cancer is low, such as Japan, incidence rates actually decline after 50 years of age [49].

It has also been reported [121] that among migrants to Israel, the shape of the age-specific incidence curve for Jews born in Europe is similar to the North American–Northern European curves, while among Asian- and African-born immigrants, the incidence rates do not increase after age 50 years. Figure 1–1 shows that in Iceland incidence rates for breast cancer have increased markedly during this century. While this increase has been taking place, the shape of the age-specific incidence curve in that country has changed from that of the "low-risk" countries to that of the "high-risk" countries [19].

Studies of Japanese-American women have indicated that there is a gradual increase in breast cancer incidence rates among descendants of migrants to Hawaii or to the mainland of the United States. Rates begin to approach those of the United States after two or three generations [31]. This suggests that environmental factors rather than genetic variables are largely responsible for the marked international differences in incidence rates.

A high-calorie or high-fat diet is one environmental factor whose distribution corresponds to the difference in incidence rates from one country to another and from one time period to another. Consistent with the role of diet is the finding that, at least in the Netherlands and Japan, incidence rates in women of lighter-than-average weight tend to plateau or decrease after age 50 to 55 years, while incidence rates in heavier women continue to increase with age [50] (see Fig. 1–1). From these data, it was concluded that perhaps half the difference in inci-

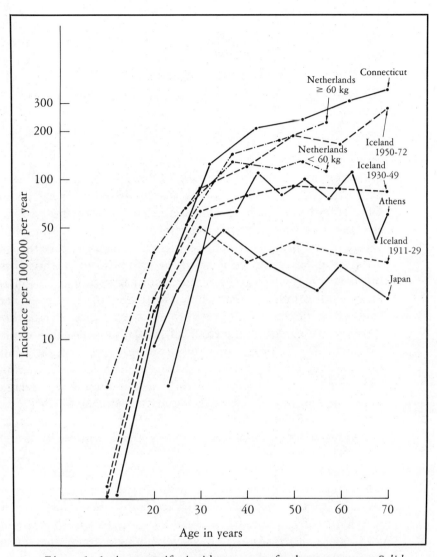

Figure 1–1. Age-specific incidence rates for breast cancer. *Solid lines:* Connecticut, USA, 1970–1974 [45]; Athens, Greece, 1966–1967 [112]; Miyagi Prefecture, Japan, 1959–1960 [52]. *Dashed lines;* Iceland, 1911–1929, Iceland, 1930–1949, Iceland, 1950–1972 [19]. *Broken lines:* Rotterdam and The Hague, the Netherlands, 1972–1974, women < 60 kg, women ≥ 60 kg [50].

dence rates between the Netherlands, where incidence rates are relatively high, and Japan, where incidence rates are low, is related to differences in the weight and height of women in these two areas. Nutrition is thus a subject of considerable interest at present and will be discussed in more detail later in this chapter.

Reproductive Variables

Early age of a woman at the birth of her first child is associated with a decreased risk for breast cancer [30, 46, 73, 97, 110, 146, 169, 184]; further, it appears that full-term pregnancies are necessary for this protective effect [98, 110, 137, 144, 186]. Women who have their first full-term pregnancy before the age of 18 years have about one-third the risk of women whose first full-term pregnancy does not occur until age 35 or older [110]. Most studies indicate that women who give birth to their first child after the age of 30 years are at an even greater risk than those who bear no children at all [110]. One possible explanation of this finding is that the protective effect of early full-term pregnancy is related to prevention of tumor initiation, while the increased risk with giving birth at older ages is related to promotion of cells that are already transformed [108].

Most investigators have found that the greater risk of breast cancer among women of low parity compared with those of high parity is attributable to the tendency of women of high parity to have given birth to their first child at a young age. While in most areas, age of the mother at the first birth does appear to account for the association of parity with breast cancer, there is evidence from studies in Burma [166], Iceland [169], and Sweden [2] that women of very high parity may in fact be protected against breast cancer independently of any association of parity with age at first birth. These recent findings merit further investigation.

The decreased risk for breast cancer among women who are relatively young at the time of the birth of their first child could be brought about by hormonal changes accompanying the pregnancy, or could be related to a factor that causes a delayed first pregnancy and also causes breast cancer. With respect to the latter possibility, it has been hypothesized that anovulatory menstrual cycles, which are associated with persistent exposure to estrogens without adequate progesterone secretion, and which would be expected to be associated with delayed first birth, could be an important risk factor for breast cancer [64, 157]. However, evidence for an etiologic role of anovulatory menstrual cycles is at present not convincing [64, 97, 165], although more research in this area is warranted. On the other hand, there is some support for the hypothesis that first birth at an early age brings about a permanent change in susceptibility; this will be discussed further in the section on endogenous hormones.

It used to be believed that breast-feeding reduced the risk for breast cancer, but this has not been found in many well-designed studies [73, 82, 97, 111, 112, 163, 166, 184]. Women with a long history of breast-feeding tend to have borne several children, and women who have borne many children tend to have had their first child at an early age. When the woman's age at first birth is taken into account, breast-feeding appears to have no effect on risk for breast cancer.

Several investigators have found that artificial menopause protects against breast cancer [46, 82, 95, 111, 146, 163]. This reduction in risk is probably attributable specifically to removal of the ovaries; and, the earlier the age at oophorectomy, the lower the risk [56, 76]. Women who undergo oophorectomy when they are below the age of 35 have about one-third the risk for breast cancer when compared to women having natural menopause around 45 to 54 years of age. This reduction in risk associated with oophorectomy appears to last for the rest of the woman's life [168].

Most studies show that menarche at an early age [30, 39, 73, 98, 137, 144, 162, 163, 166, 169, 186], and menopause at a late age [30, 39, 73, 98, 137, 163, 166, 168, 184, 186] are associated with an increased risk for breast cancer. It is not known whether a woman's risk is directly affected by the total number of years she has menstrual cycles, or whether age at menarche and age at menopause are important risk factors in their own right, regardless of the number of years of menstrual activity.

Endogenous Hormones

The results of epidemiologic studies clearly suggest that hormones are involved in the etiology of breast cancer. Despite a large amount of laboratory and epidemiologic research, however, there is still great uncertainty as to which hormones are involved and in what manner they have their effects. The hormones that have been most frequently considered in the etiology of breast cancer are estrogens, progesterone, prolactin, androgens, and thyroid hormones.

Estrogens

Estrogens have long been considered possible mammary carcinogens in women because of (1) the epidemiologic characteristics of breast cancer; (2) evidence that estrogens are carcinogenic in animals, particularly in the tumor promotion stage; and (3) evidence that some tumors respond to the administration of estrogenic or antiestrogenic compounds. The relatively long period of time over which risk factors related to estrogens have their effect suggests that estrogens are involved in tumor initiation, regardless of what role they may have in tumor promotion [107]. It has been noted [44], however, that any simple explanation based on total exposure to estrogens is unlikely since full-term pregnancies at an early age, when estrogen levels are increased, are in fact associated with decreased risk for breast cancer; and, also, there is no decreased risk associated with lactation, when exposure to cyclic estrogens is suppressed.

It was hypothesized by Lemon and co-workers [93], and subsequently in modified form by Cole and MacMahon [44], that the roles of the three main types of estrogens—estrone (E1), estradiol (E2), and estriol (E3)—need to be considered. Cole and MacMahon proposed that the greater the amount of estriol (E3) relative to estrone and estradiol that a women produces during the years immediately after menarche, the lower her lifetime risk of breast cancer. This hypothesis was consistent with the finding from epidemiologic studies that full-term pregnancies protect against breast cancer, since during the third trimester of pregnancy, concentrations of estriol increase greatly relative to estrone and estradiol. This hypothesis was also supported by certain animal experiments which indicated that (1) estrone and estradiol were carcinogenic in certain animals while estriol was, at most, weakly carcinogenic; (2) estriol competed with estradiol for cytoplasmic binding sites; and (3) estriol inhibited the incorporation of estradiol into nuclei of a chemically induced rat tumor [44]. A variety of circumstantial epidemiologic evidence has subsequently supported this hypothesis. In two reports, for instance, it was found that the estriol ratio (E3/[E1 + E2]), as determined from urine specimens, was higher in young Asian women than in young North American women [109], and that young Japanese and Chinese women in Hawaii had estriol ratios intermediate between their counterparts living in Japan and in the mainland United States [51]. Also, it was reported in a study from Israel that the estriol ratio was higher in urine samples from migrants to Israel who had come from countries with low incidence rates of breast cancer than that found in migrants from countries with high rates of breast cancer [66].

Despite these and other circumstantial pieces of epidemiologic evidence, the hypothesis that a high ratio of estriol to estrone and estradiol protects against breast cancer has been criticized for several reasons. It is known, for instance, that only small amounts of estriol enter the blood; estriol is concentrated in the urine, and urine concentrations are not indicative of blood concentrations [99, 101]. It has been reported, too, that estriol does not effectively compete with estradiol in mammary tumors of patients undergoing mastectomy [48], that estriol is bound only weakly to receptor sites [9], and that estriol does promote uterine growth in a manner similar to estradiol. Furthermore, it has been found that tumors in mice can be produced by estriol [143].

Thus, although there is much circumstantial evidence to support the estriol ratio hypothesis, it is still the subject of much debate. Most investigators would appear to agree with Longcope and Pratt [101], who suggest that the estriol ratio in the urine may be an indicator of risk. It probably is not indicative of amounts of biologically active estrogens in the blood but reflects differences in metabolic pathways, which perhaps could be of more direct causal significance.

The etiologic role of estrone has also been a subject of interest. Estrone is known to be carcinogenic in animals, would tend to be at high concentrations when the estriol ratio is low, and is believed to be involved in the etiology of endometrial cancer when it is unopposed by progesterone. In postmenopausal women, most circulating estrogen occurs in the form of estrone [136]. The conversion from its precursor androstenedione occurs in adipose tissue [148, 160], and thus obesity is associated with increased conversion of androstenedione to estrone [65]. For this reason, then, a role for estrone in the etiology of breast cancer occurring postmenopausally would be consistent with obesity as a risk factor and hence with a role for diet. Although it is known that severe undernutrition causes a decrease in the urinary excretion of all the urinary estrogens and the estriol ratio [188], there is no direct evidence of effects on estrogens of more subtle differences in nutrition.

Progesterone

The role of progesterone in the etiology of breast cancer has not been so well studied. Progesterone has been found to be a cocarcinogen in rodents [123, 134], but more attention has been focused on its possible protective effect against estrogens. It has been hypothesized [157] that estrogenic stimulation in the absence of sufficient progesterone secretion may provide a favorable environment for the development of breast cancer. Postmenopausal production of estrone without progesterone could thus be postulated to be associated with an increase in risk. It was mentioned earlier that the evidence is unclear as to whether anovulatory cycles in the years following menarche, with their exposures to estrogens without adequate levels of progesterone, increase the risk for breast cancer. Thus, the role of progesterone in the etiology of breast cancer and of the way it interacts with estrogens and other hormones is an area of continued research interest.

Prolactin

It has been found that prolactin participates both in the initiation and promotion of mammary tumors in mice and rats. It is also known that there are complex interactions among prolactin, estrogens, and progesterone as well as other hormones [123, 147], so it is difficult to determine the specific effects of prolactin. Although some investigators [72, 133] have found higher prolactin concentrations (and also estrogen concentrations) in the daughters of women with breast cancer than in the daughters of controls, there is in general little evidence that prolactin plays an important role in the etiology of breast cancer in humans. Prolactin levels have been found to be similar in populations at both high and low risk for breast cancer [75, 89]. Also, it has been pointed out by MacMahon, Cole, and Brown [108] that prolactin is elevated in normal women only during pregnancies and lactation, yet lactation has no effect on breast cancer risk and full-term pregnancies are protective. Thus, evidence of a major role for prolactin in the etiology of human breast cancer is at present weak.

Thyroid Hormones

In respect to thyroid hormones, it has been reported that (1) areas that have had high rates of goiter have high mortality rates for breast cancer [24], (2) patients with breast cancer have a higher than expected frequency of hypothyroidism [15, 24, 184], and (3) patients with hyperthyroidism are unlikely to develop breast cancer [78]. On closer examination, however, those studies at most provide only slight support for such an association, and Kirschner [86] has concluded that no unified hypothesis has been proposed to date to relate thyroid function to risk of breast cancer.

No definite risk indicators among the hormones or among combinations of hormones have been found, but the most promising leads involve the estrogens and the possible interactions of estrogens with other hormones. So much data suggests that hormones do play a central role in breast cancer etiology that the role of hormones certainly should be the subject of a great deal of research. It nevertheless is a particularly hard area for study because of the difficulties of measurement, the variation of hormone concentrations in a given individual from one time to another, the interrelationships among the hormones, and the probable need to measure hormones long before breast cancer develops.

Exogenous Hormones

The likelihood that endogenous hormones are involved in breast cancer etiology has generated considerable interest in the possible etiologic involvement of exogenous hormones, particularly those that contain estrogens. The oral contraceptives that have been marketed to date contain either estradiol or a chemically similar compound, mestranol, in combination with various progesterones, while the most widely used form of estrogen replacement therapy contains estrone and no progesterones.

Oral Contraceptives

There is little evidence at present that oral contraceptives either increase or decrease the risk for breast cancer [83, 128, 141, 146, 170, 171]. In certain studies, however, increased risks have been reported among certain subgroups of women, including (1) women who have taken oral contraceptives for relatively long periods of time and who have had biopsy-confirmed benign breast disease prior to the development of the carcinoma [30, 129], and (2) women who have used oral contraceptives before their first pregnancy [129]. Until these results are evaluated in other studies, however, it is not known whether these findings occurred by chance or whether they suggest a tendency of oral contraceptives to enhance the effect of certain other risk factors. In any event, it is generally agreed that if oral contraceptives affect the initiation of breast tumors, this effect probably would not be observable until a latent period of perhaps 15 to 20 years had elapsed from the time they were first used. Since oral contraceptives were first approved for use in the United States in 1960 and in other western countries at about the same time, findings over the next few years will be critical.

Several epidemiologic studies, however, have indicated that use of oral contraceptives for 2 to 4 or more years is associated with a decreased frequency of fibrocystic disease and fibroadenomas of the breast [28, 55, 128, 141, 145, 171, 172]. In one study [142] it was found that the progesterone content of the pill was responsible for the decrease in risk.

Thus, long-term oral contraceptive use is associated with a decreased frequency of benign breast diseases but, on the basis of current evidence, does not appear to decrease the risk for breast cancer. On the other hand, fibrocystic disease and possibly fibroadenoma are associated with an increased risk for breast cancer. To resolve this apparent paradox it has been hypothesized [43] that the forms of benign breast disease against which oral contraceptives appear to protect may be different from the forms associated with a high risk for breast cancer. In fact, it was recently reported [100] that long-term oral contraceptive use was negatively associated with fibrocystic disease only in patients with no or minimal ductal atypia as graded by the Black-Chabon system [21]. If this finding is confirmed in other studies, it would have implications for breast cancer risk among oral contraceptive users, since the forms of fibrocystic disease most strongly associated with breast cancer [20, 87] were not the forms for which long-term contraceptive users showed a lower frequency of occurrence [100]. It is also possible that oral contraceptive use is in some way impeding clinical recognition of fibrocystic disease with no or minimal ductal atypia.

Conjugated Estrogens

Although some studies [30, 33, 34, 146, 175, 179] have found no increased risk or even a reduced risk for breast cancer among women using conjugated estrogens during and following menopause, most of these studies have serious methodological limitations, for example, small sample size, short period of follow-up, and inadequate comparison groups. In one study [37], the possibility of an adverse effect was raised when age at natural menopause and age at diagnosis were both taken into account. In a second study [77] with a relatively long period of follow-up, an increased risk for breast cancer was observed in women who had first used estrogen replacement therapy 10 to 15 years previously. In the second study [77], the risk for breast cancer was found to be particularly high among women in whom benign breast disease developed after they had started using conjugated estrogens, a finding similar to that mentioned earlier for the breast cancer risk among women who had a history both of benign breast disease and long-term contraceptive use [30, 129].

An association between conjugated estrogens and breast cancer would be consistent with the hypothesis that estrone (or estrone unopposed by progesterones) is carcinogenic to breast tissue, since estrone is the type of estrogen found in the most widely used estrogen replacement compound. At present, however, it is uncertain whether estrogen replacement therapy does alter the risk for breast cancer. What is needed is further study in which the probably long latent period is taken into account and in which women with and without known benign breast disease are considered separately.

Diethylstilbestrol and Thyroid Hormone Therapy

The possibility of an increased risk for breast cancer among women who were previously exposed to diethylstilbestrol during their pregnancy or pregnancies has been suggested by one study [18], although the number of cases in this study was too small for definitive conclusions to be reached.

Finally, an initial report [81] of an increased risk of breast cancer among women who have had thyroid hormone therapy was not verified in subsequent studies [30, 124, 174].

Diet

Experiments in rats and mice have shown that a high-fat diet with or without certain mammary carcinogens is associated with an increase in the number of mammary tumors, and that this is not attributable to total caloric intake or various other dietary constituents [35, 61]. Furthermore, there is a fairly strong correlation between the per capita consumption of fats and oils and breast cancer mortality rates in countries for which these data are available [11, 36]. This correlation is higher for fats than for other dietary constituents or for other more direct indicators of socioeconomic status [11, 54, 70].

A variety of other circumstantial evidence also suggests an etiologic role for dietary fat. An increase in breast cancer death rates among offspring of Japanese migrants to the United States [31] has occurred as their dietary habits have changed. Within England, a positive correlation between dietary fat consumption and breast cancer mortality rates has been reported [164]. Breast cancer death rates are low for Seventh-Day Adventists, who have a relatively low fat intake [132]. Also, an increase in breast cancer incidence and mortality has occurred in Iceland as the diet has become more westernized [19, 119]. These studies, however, by no means provide definitive evidence for a causal role of diet, since other socioeconomic variables might also explain these trends. Studies comparing previous dietary habits of breast cancer patients and other women of similar age have been only slightly suggestive of an association of a high-fat diet with risk for breast cancer [120, 132]; it must be realized, however, that obtaining reliable dietary data is extremely difficult, and there is not a great deal of variation in dietary habits within study populations. Thus, although a role for a high-fat diet in the etiology of human breast cancer remains an attractive hypothesis, definitive evidence is difficult to obtain.

Various mechanisms have been suggested to account for an effect of diet on risk for breast cancer. Perhaps the most reasonable hypothesis [42] is that a diet with excess caloric intake increases the amount of adipose tissue, which in turn influences hormonal levels, such as the amount of circulating estrone; these altered hormonal levels could then influence the risk for breast cancer. It is not clear, however, why diets high in fat would have a greater effect by this mechanism than would other types of high-calorie diets. It is also possible that diet affects breast cancer risk by its influence on age at menarche [1, 60].

Familial Aggregation and Genetics

In women who have a first-degree relative with breast cancer the risk for breast cancer is two to three times the risk in the general population [6, 105, 167]. It is not known to what extent genetic factors or exposure to similar environmental agents are responsible for this elevated risk.

In some families genetic factors appear to be very important. Lynch and Krush [102], for example, have reported that in a few families the risk to first-degree relatives approaches 50 percent, a figure consistent with autosómal dominant inheritance. In general, it is believed that the postulated genetic effect is more important when cases in relatives occur premenopausally rather than postmenopausally and is more important when there are bilateral carcinomas as opposed to unilateral carcinoma [5, 6, 8, 58]. Anderson [5–7] has found that the risk for breast cancer in first-degree relatives is increased threefold if the patient with carcinoma is premenopausal, but only by a factor of 1.5 if the patient is postmenopausal. He found a fivefold increase in risk for women with first-degree relatives who had bilateral disease but very little increase in risk if the first-degree relative had unilateral disease. For women who had first-degree relatives with postmenopausal and bilateral breast cancer, the risk was increased by a factor of four, but if the disease in the first-degree relative was bilateral and occurred premenopausally, there was almost a ninefold increase in risk.

In addition, Anderson [7] has found that if both a mother and a sister have had breast cancer, the risk is much higher than if only the sister has had breast cancer. In families in which bilateral disease has occurred premenopausally in both the mother and the sister, the risk of breast cancer for other daughters is estimated to be 30 percent before they reach 40 years of age.

Anderson [7] has also found that susceptibility to breast cancer is just as likely to occur through paternal lines of descent as through maternal lines.

In conclusion, although a few families appear to have a strong genetic predisposition to breast cancer, and although heredity probably does play a role in premenopausal and bilateral disease, most of the known epidemiologic characteristics of breast cancer are probably related to environmental rather than to hereditary factors [108].

Benign Breast Diseases

Women with diagnosed fibrocystic breast disease have about a twofold to fourfold increase in risk for subsequent breast cancer [47, 53, 67, 68, 87, 94, 122, 135]. This elevated risk has been found to persist for at least 30 years after the diagnosis of fibrocystic disease [122]. Evidence that fibroadenoma of the breast increases the risk for breast cancer is less strong [53, 94, 135], but in one recent longitudinal study [87], there was a marked elevation in risk. Furthermore, this follow-up study [87] found that women with a history of fibroadenoma were particularly likely to develop adenocarcinoma of the breast, while women with fibrocystic breast disease were more likely to be affected with infiltrating duct carcinoma. In any event, fibrocystic disease has been studied more extensively than fibroadenoma, probably because it is much more common and tends to occur in an older age group; these factors make its relationship to breast cancer less difficult to study than that of fibroadenoma.

It is likely that the various forms of fibrocystic disease are associated with different risks for breast cancer. Haagensen [67, 68], who has classified cases of fibrocystic disease according to histologic patterns, has reported that multiple duct papillomas, gross cystic disease, and lobular neoplasia (lobular carcinoma in situ) predispose a woman to breast cancer. A specific correlation between large duct hyperplasia and subsequent cancer of the breast has been suggested by Humphrey and Swerdlow [79]. McDivitt and associates [113] reported from a longitudinal study that in-situ lobular carcinoma is a preinvasive form of infiltrating lobular carcinoma and is associated with a high risk for cancer in the opposite breast as well.

Black and colleagues [20, 21] have suggested a method of quantifying epithelial breast lesions and reported that the risk for breast cancer varies according to the degree of atypia and hyperplasia seen in the benign mammary epithelium. This finding was confirmed by Kodlin and associates [87] in a follow-up study of women with all types of benign breast diseases. Page and co-workers [130], on the other hand, have found that epithelial proliferative lesions involving ductal hyperplasia, papillary epithelial hyperplasia with cytologic apocrine-like changes, and lobular hyperplasia are all associated with an elevated risk for breast cancer; they also found that the extent of atypia in the ductal epithelial cells does not provide any further information on breast cancer risk. Given these somewhat contradictory reports, it would be desirable for other investigators to examine the relative importance of hyperplasia and atypia, and of ductal and lobular lesions in predicting the development of breast cancer. Although systems of nomenclature and classification of fibrocystic disease differ among pathologists, it appears that in all systems of classification epithelial disturbances of some type are associated with an increased risk for breast cancer.

The biologic basis for the relationship between fibrocystic disease and breast cancer is unknown. Fibrocystic disease may be a premalignant condition. Autopsy studies [59, 161] clearly show that fibrocystic disease may be present in several parts of the breast of women who have not sought care for breast disease. Thus, it is possible that premalignant cells are dispersed throughout the breasts of some women with fibrocystic disease, and that the diagnosed cystic disease may only be the most obvious part of a widely dispersed pathologic process; on the other hand, an abnormal hormonal milieu could exist in some women with fibrocystic disease that makes all breast epithelial cells "premalignant" or susceptible to a carcinogenic agent.

Multiple Primary Cancers Involving the Breast and Other Sites

Women with cancer in one breast have four to five times the risk of women of comparable age in the general population of having a second primary cancer in the other breast [140, 150, 151]. Various investigators have reported that multiple primary cancers involving the breast, endometrium, and ovary also occur more frequently than would be expected by chance [106, 138, 149, 151, 152, 173]. In general, women who have cancer in one of these three sites have about twice the risk for cancer in another of these sites, although the elevation in risk varies somewhat from one site to another. There is also some evidence of an excess of multiple primary cancers involving the breast and colon, but the evidence for such an association is not entirely consistent [149, 151, 152].

Mortality for breast, ovarian, and colon cancers in various countries around the world are correlated [185]. Within the United States high mortality for breast cancer, colon cancer, ovarian cancer, and to a certain extent endometrial cancer, tends to be found in the same regions of the country [22, 32].

It has been suggested that the reason for the higher than expected frequency of these multiple primary cancers in individuals and for the correlation among the mortality and incidence rates for these cancers in various geographic areas is that certain individuals and certain localities may have high levels of exposure to etiologic agents common to more than one of these cancers, for example, a high-fat diet, particular hormonal patterns, or reduced fertility [92, 149, 150]. Within an individual the presence of one tumor may predispose to another. For instance, an ovarian tumor may be responsible for an increased risk for breast cancer because of higher levels of hormone secreted from the ovary.

Radiation

It is known that radiation to the chest in high doses can cause breast cancer. Evidence comes from follow-up studies of survivors of the atomic bombs in Japan [80, 114, 177], of women undergoing radiation treatment for acute postpartum mastitis [118, 158], and of women who underwent fluoroscopy in the course of treatment of tuberculosis by pneumothorax [26, 104, 125]. Animal studies also clearly indicate an association between radiation and breast cancer [38]. The report of the Advisory Committee on the Biological Effects of Ionizing Radiation (BEIR) [3] for the National Academy of Sciences–National Research Council estimated that in North America the risk for breast cancer is about 6 cases/10^6 women/year/rad, which corresponds to a doubling of the risk of breast cancer with exposure to 120 rads, or a 0.83 percent increase per rad over the incidence rate that would have occurred otherwise.

Radiation may have a particularly marked effect in women who were exposed between the ages of 10 to 19 years [25, 26, 114, 125]. The risk appears to be greatest if the exposure occurred just before and during menarche [27], suggesting that at this period of life the breast tissue is especially sensitive to radiation. Two reasons for this increased sensitivity might be that the breasts are rapidly developing during this period of life, or that most women have not given birth to their first child at this time and the breasts may be more susceptible before the first birth occurs [114]. Exposure of the breast to radiation during a woman's first pregnancy has also been found to confer greater risk than exposures before or after the first pregnancy, suggesting that indeed the breasts are most susceptible to the carcinogenic effects of radiation at a time of high mitotic activity such as around the time of menarche and during pregnancy [27]. To date, women exposed to radiation before the age of 10 years show no increased risk for breast cancer, but most of these women have not yet entered the age group at high risk for breast cancer.

It has also recently been found that multiple exposures to low doses have a cumulative effect, so that the risk of several small exposures is about the same as the effect of one large dose of the same magnitude [25, 26, 158]. The effects of radiation appear to be permanent and are still apparent for as long as exposed women have been followed [26, 158]. Although there are data available on increased risks at very low levels of exposure to radiation, it has been found that among atomic bomb survivors, exposure to radiation somewhat under 50 rads is associated with an increased risk for breast cancer [90]. It is felt by many investigators [25, 26, 114, 158] that a linear dose-response relationship provides a reasonably good fit to the available data.

Exposure to Radiation in Screening for Breast Cancer

Bailar [16], in a paper published in 1976, raised the question of whether the low doses of radiation to which women are exposed while undergoing mammography in screening programs could actually increase the risk of breast cancer. Since the shape of the dose-response curve at low levels is not definitely known, no certain answer to this question can be given. Also, only recently have large numbers of women undergone mammography, so a carcinogenic effect would probably not yet be detectable. However, the finding [25, 90] that an increase in risk is detectable following exposure to only moderate doses and the belief [25, 26, 114, 158] that a linear dose-response relationship provides a reasonable fit to the data have justified a certain amount of concern. Furthermore, results from a randomized trial done at the Health Insurance Plan (HIP) of Greater New York indicated that periodic screening in women under 50 years of age brought about no demonstrable saving of lives, whereas in women over 50 years of age, a definite decrease in breast cancer mortality was attributable to screening [156]. Mammography was one component of the overall screening, and it has been estimated that its contribution to the overall beneficial effect occurring in women over age 50 is likely to be on the order of 20 to 33 percent [17, 156].

After considering the various pieces of evidence on the benefits and risks from screening by means of mammography, the National Cancer Institute ad hoc groups [126] reached the following conclusions: (1) mammography probably does at least slightly increase the risk for breast cancer; (2) the doses of radiation in mammography should therefore be reduced as much as possible; (3) since the benefits from mammography have not been shown to occur in women below the age of 50 years, the use of mammography in routine screening in these younger women should be stopped; and (4) further randomized trials should be undertaken in women over 50 years of age.

Because mammographic techniques have improved considerably in recent years, mammography may now detect with greater accuracy lesions in breasts of premenopausal women. It is thus possible that the failure of the HIP study to find screening beneficial in women under 50 years of age would not occur in a study done now [156, 178]. Also, if radiation is an important risk factor for breast cancer primarily for females at quite young ages, then possibly the lower limit for screening of women by mammography could be reduced to as low as 30 years of age.

Mammographic Parenchymal Patterns

Wolfe [180–183] has reported that breast parenchymal patterns seen on xeromammograms can be useful in predicting risks for breast cancer. He has divided breast parenchyma into four types: N1, essentially normal breast composed mostly of fat with no ducts visible; P1, parenchyma mostly fat with some prominent ducts occupying up to one quarter the volume of the breast; P2, similar to P1 but with prominent ducts occupying more than one quarter the volume of the breast; and DY, extremely dense, dysplastic parenchyma, which usually denotes connective tissue hyperplasia. Several investigators [88, 131, 178], but not all [117, 139], have found that in women under the age of 50 years, DY patterns are associated with a substantial increase in the frequency of occurrence of breast cancer, and that P2, and possibly P1, patterns are associated with a moderate elevation in frequency. Additional longitudinal studies are needed to evaluate Wolfe's findings further.

Viruses

The presence of a mammary tumor virus in mice has naturally brought about a great deal of interest in the possibility of a viral etiology for human breast cancer. However, the evidence for and against the role of viruses in the etiology of human breast cancer has been reviewed by MacMahon, Cole, and Brown [108] and Henderson [71], who could find no convincing evidence for a viral etiology. Even in susceptible mice, there is evidence that estrogen stimulation may be necessary for the mouse mammary tumor virus to produce tumors [63]. Although it is certainly still possible that viruses are involved, at present there is little evidence to support this view.

Other "Exposures" of Current Interest

Reserpine

In three epidemiologic studies [13, 29, 69] published in the same issue of the *Lancet* in 1974, a causal association between use of the antihypertensive drug reserpine and the development of breast cancer was suggested. A plausible biologic explanation was the prolactin-stimulating property of reserpine [29]. These studies were subject to immediate criticism on methodological grounds. Subsequent results from several more epidemiologic studies [12, 14, 40, 84, 91, 96, 103, 127] have not supported the original findings. With one possible exception [12] they have indicated that there is at most only a slight association between reserpine and breast cancer. Thus, unless more convincing evidence is presented to the contrary, epidemiologic studies do not provide much support for the hypothesis that use of reserpine increases the risk for breast cancer, although it should be recognized that in epidemiologic studies it is difficult to determine whether slight associations are causal or incidental. The strong or even moderate associations that were originally reported [13, 29, 69], however, are almost certainly overestimates of any true association.

Hair Dyes
There has also been interest in whether exposure to hair dyes increases the risk for cancers. This interest seems to stem from reports that many permanent and semipermanent hair dyes are mutagenic in bacterial test systems [4, 153]. Epidemiologic studies of hairdressers and of women who dye their own hair have produced somewhat conflicting results [74, 85, 116, 155, 159, 176], but the majority indicate that there is no increase in risk for breast cancer among women who dye their hair or who are exposed to hair dyes professionally. However, it is still possible, but perhaps unlikely, that certain subgroups of women are at high risk if they dye their hair. Further epidemiologic studies that are carefully designed specifically to test the hypothesis about hair dyes are needed before any definite conclusions can be reached.

Table 1–1 summarizes the current state of knowledge of risk factors for breast cancer. The strongest risk factors are increasing age, a history of bilateral breast cancer occurring premenopausally in a first-degree relative, a history of breast cancer in one breast, and residence from an early age in North America or northern Europe. Other risk factors—including whether or not a woman has had her ovaries removed, age at first birth, a history of benign breast disease, previous exposure to relatively high levels of radiation in the chest such as occurred in the treatment of postpartum mastitis and tuberculosis, a history of

Table 1-1 Summary of Risk Factors for Breast Cancer.

Variable	Factors Associated with High Risk	Factors Associated with Low Risk
Greater than fourfold differential in risk		
Age	Old age	Young age
Family history of bilateral breast cancer occurring premenopausally	Present	Absent
History of cancer in one breast	Present	Absent
Country of residence at early age	North America, northern Europe	Asia, Africa
Twofold to fourfold differential in risk		
Oophorectomy	Ovaries intact	Ovaries removed
Age at birth of first child	Older than 30	Younger than 30
History of benign breast disease	Present	Absent
Amount of radiation to chest	Large doses	Minimal doses
History of any first-degree relative with breast cancer	Present	Absent
Postmenopausal body build	Heavy	Thin
Socioeconomic class	Upper	Lower
History of primary cancer in ovary or endometrium	Present	Absent
Less than twofold differential in risk		
Age at menarche	Early	Late
Age at menopause	Late	Early
Marital status	Never married	Married now or at one time
Place of residence	Urban	Rural
Race	White	Black

breast cancer in any first-degree relative, obesity, high socio-economic status, and a previous cancer in the ovaries or endometrium—are associated with elevations in risk ranging from twofold to fourfold. Finally, age at menarche, age at menopause, marital status, place of residence, and race—white as compared to black—are associated with small but real differentials in risk.

The majority of these factors contribute only moderately to the risk for breast cancer. Thus, our current state of knowledge suggests that for most women many variables act together to determine risk for breast cancer. Whether several of these can be related to some underlying mechanism such as a particular hormonal profile is not yet known. Also, it may be noted that most of the risk factors identified so far are not readily amenable to preventive measures. Nevertheless, knowledge of breast cancer epidemiology has been gradually evolving over the years, and various leads for further research are available. Although feasible ways of substantially reducing the high incidence of breast cancer are not yet known, the magnitude of the problem clearly indicates that this is an important area for study.

References

1. Acheson, R. M. Maturation of the Skeleton. In F. Faulkner (Ed.), *Human Development*. Philadelphia: Saunders, 1966.
2. Adami, H. O., Rimsten, A., Stenkvist, B., et al. Reproductive history and breast cancer. *Cancer* 41:747, 1978.
3. Advisory Committee on the Biological Effects of Ionizing Radiation. *Report on the Effects on Population of Exposure to Low Levels of Ionizing Radiation*. Washington, D.C.: National Academy of Sciences–National Research Council, 1972.
4. Ames, B. N., Kammen, H. O., and Yamasaki, E. Hair dyes are mutagenic: Identification of a variety of mutagenic ingredients. *Proc. Natl. Acad. Sci. U.S.A.* 72:2423, 1972.
5. Anderson, D. E. Some characteristics of familial breast cancer. *Cancer* 28:1500, 1971.
6. Anderson, D. E. A genetic study of human breast cancer. *J. Natl. Cancer Inst.* 48:1029, 1972.
7. Anderson, D. E. Genetic study of breast cancer: Identification of a high risk group. *Cancer* 34:1090, 1974.
8. Anderson, D. E. Breast cancer in families. *Cancer* 40:1855, 1977.
9. Anderson, J. N., Peck, E. J., and Clark, J. H. Estrogen-induced uterine responses and growth: Relationship to receptor estrogen binding by uterine necks. *Endocrinology* 96:160, 1975.
10. Armstrong, B. Recent trends in breast cancer incidence and

mortality in relation to changes in possible risk factors. *Int. J. Cancer* 17:204, 1976.

11. Armstrong, B., and Doll, R. Environmental factors and cancer incidence and mortality in different countries with special reference to dietary practices. *Int. J. Cancer* 15:617, 1975.

12. Armstrong, B., Skegg, D., White, G., et al. Rauwolfia derivatives and breast cancer in hypertensive women. *Lancet* 2:8, 1976.

13. Armstrong, B., Stevens, N., and Doll, R. Retrospective study of the association between use of rauwolfia derivatives and breast cancer in English women. *Lancet* 2:672, 1974.

14. Aromaa, A., Hakama, M., Hakulinen, T., et al. Breast cancer and use of rauwolfia and other antihypertensive agents in hypertensive patients: A nationwide case-control study in Finland. *Int. J. Cancer* 18:727, 1976.

15. Backwinkel, K., and Jackson, A. S. Some features of breast cancer and thyroid deficiency. *Cancer* 17:1174, 1964.

16. Bailar, J. C., III. Mammography: A contrary view. *Ann. Intern. Med.* 84:77, 1976.

17. Bailar, J.C., III. Screening for early breast cancer: Pros and cons. *Cancer* 39:2783, 1977.

18. Bibbo, M., Haenszel, W. M., Wied, G. L., et al. A twenty-five year follow-up study of women exposed to diethylstilbestrol during pregnancy. *N. Engl. J. Med.* 298:763, 1978.

19. Bjarnason, O., Day, N., Snaedal, G., et al. The effect of year of birth on the breast cancer age-incidence curve in Iceland. *Int. J. Cancer* 13:689, 1974.

20. Black, M. M., Barclay, T. H. C., Cutler, S. J., et al. Association of atypical characteristics of benign breast lesions with subsequent risk of breast cancer. *Cancer* 29:338, 1972.

21. Black, M. M., Chabon, A. B. In situ carcinoma of the breast. *Pathol. Annu.* 4:185, 1969.

22. Blot, W. J., Fraumeni, J. F., Jr., Stone, B. J. Geographic patterns of breast cancer in the United States. *J. Natl. Cancer Inst.* 59:1407, 1977.

23. Blot, W. J., Fraumeni, J. F., Jr., and Young, J. L., Jr. Left-sided breast cancer. *Lancet* 2:762, 1977.

24. Bogardus, G. M., and Finley, J. W. Breast cancer and thyroid disease. *Surgery* 49:461, 1961.

25. Boice, J. D., Jr., Land, C. E., Shore, R. E., et al. Risk of breast cancer following low-dose radiation exposure. *Radiology* 131:589, 1979.

26. Boice, J. D., Jr., and Monson, R. R. Breast cancer in women after repeated fluoroscopic examinations of the chest. *J. Natl. Cancer Inst.* 59:823, 1977.

27. Boice, J. D., Jr., and Stone, B. J. Interaction Between Radiation and Other Breast Cancer Risk Factors. In *Late Biological Effects of Ionizing Radiation,* Vol. I. Vienna: International Atomic Energy Agency, 1978. Pp. 231–249.

28. Boston Collaborative Drug Surveillance Program. Oral contraceptives and venous thromboembolic disease, surgically confirmed gallbladder disease, and breast tumours. *Lancet* 1:1399, 1973.

29. Boston Collaborative Drug Surveillance Program. Reserpine and breast cancer. *Lancet* 2:669, 1974.

30. Brinton, L. A., Williams, R. R., Hoover, R. N., et al. Breast cancer risk factors among screening program participants. *J. Natl. Cancer Inst.* 62:37, 1979.

31. Buell, P. Changing incidence of breast cancer in Japanese-American women. *J. Natl. Cancer Inst.* 51:1479, 1973.

32. Burbank, F. A sequential space-time cluster analysis of cancer mortality in the United States: Etiologic implications. *Am. J. Epidemiol.* 95:393, 1972.

33. Burch, J. C., and Byrd, B. F., Jr. Effects of long-term administration of estrogen in the occurrence of mammary cancer in women. *Ann. Surg.* 174:414, 1971.

34. Burch, J. C., Byrd, B. F., Jr., and Vaughn, W. K. The effects of long-term estrogen on hysterectomized women. *Am. J. Obstet. Gynecol.* 118:778, 1974.

35. Carroll, K. K. Experimental evidence of dietary factors and hormone dependent cancers. *Cancer Res.* 35:3374, 1975.

36. Carroll, K. K., Gammel, E. B., and Plunkett, E. R. Dietary fat and mammary cancer. *Can. Med. Assoc. J.* 98:590, 1968.

37. Casagrande, J., Gerkins, V., Henderson, B. E., et al. Exogenous estrogens and breast cancer in women with natural menopause. *J. Natl. Cancer Inst.* 56:839, 1976.

38. Casarett, G. W. Experimental radiation carcinogenesis. *Prog. Exp. Tumor Res.* 7:48, 1965.

39. Choi, N. W., Howe, G. R., Miller, A. B., et al. An epidemiologic study of breast cancer. *Am. J. Epidemiol.* 107:510, 1978.

40. Christopher, L. J., Crooks, J., Davidson, J. F., et al. A multicentre study of rauwolfia derivates and breast cancer. *Eur. J. Clin. Pharmacol.* 11:409, 1977.

41. Cohart, E. Socioeconomic distribution of cancer of the female sex organs in New Haven. *Cancer* 8:34, 1955.

42. Cole, P., and Cramer, D. Diet and cancer of the endocrine target organs. *Cancer* 40(Suppl. 1):434, 1977.

43. Cole, P., Elwood, J. M., and Kaplan, S. D. Incidence rates and risk factors of benign breast neoplasms. *Am. J. Epidemiol.* 108:112, 1978.

44. Cole, P., and MacMahon, B. Oestrogen fractions during early reproductive life in the aetiology of breast cancer. *Lancet* 1:604, 1969.

45. Connecticut Tumor Registry. Unpublished data, 1979.

46. Craig, T. J., Comstock, G. W., and Geiser, P. B. Epidemiologic comparison of breast cancer patients with early and late onset of malignancy and general population controls. *J. Natl. Cancer Inst.* 53:1577, 1974.

47. Davis, H. H., Simons, M., and Davis, J. B. Cystic disease of the breast: Relationship to carcinoma. *Cancer* 17:957, 1964.
48. Deshpande, N., Carson, P., and Horner, J. Oestriol in human breast tumours. *J. Steroid Biochem.* 7:11, 1976.
49. DeWaard, F. The epidemiology of breast cancer: Review and prospects. *Int. J. Cancer* 4:577, 1969.
50. DeWaard, F., Cornelis, J. P., Aoki, K., et al. Breast cancer incidence according to weight and height in two cities of the Netherlands and in Aichi Prefective, Japan. *Cancer* 40:1269, 1977.
51. Dickinson, L. E., MacMahon, B., Cole, P., et al. Estrogen profiles of oriental and caucasian women in Hawaii. *N. Engl. J. Med.* 291:1211, 1974.
52. Doll, R., Payne, P., and Waterhouse, J. *Cancer Incidence in Five Continents.* Berlin: Springer-Verlag, 1966.
53. Donnelly, P. K., Baker, K. W., Carney, J. A., et al. Benign breast lesions and subsequent breast carcinoma in Rochester, Minnesota. *Mayo Clin. Proc.* 50:650, 1975.
54. Drasar, B. S., and Irving, D. Environmental factors and cancer of the colon and breast. *Br. J. Cancer* 27:167, 1973.
55. Fasal, E., and Paffenbarger, R. S. Oral contraceptives as related to cancer and benign lesions of the breast. *J. Natl. Cancer Inst.* 55:767, 1975.
56. Feinleib, M. Breast cancer and artificial menopause: A cohort study. *J. Natl. Cancer Inst.* 41:315, 1968.
57. Feinleib, M., and Garrison, R. J. Interpretation of the vital statistics of breast cancer. *Cancer* 24:1109, 1969.
58. Finney, G. G., Jr., Finney, G. G., Montague, A. C. W., et al. Bilateral breast cancer; clinical and pathological review. *Ann. Surg.* 175:635, 1972.
59. Frantz, V. K., Pickren, J. W., Melcher, G. W., et al. Incidence of chronic cystic disease in so-called "normal breasts": A study based on 225 postmortem examinations. *Cancer* 4:762, 1951.
60. Frisch, R. E. Critical Weight at Menarche, Initiation of the Adolescent Growth Spurt, and Control of Puberty. In M. M. Grumbach, G. D. Grave, and F. E. Mayer (Eds.), *Control of the Onset of Puberty.* New York: Wiley, 1974.
61. Gammal, E. B., Carroll, K. K., and Plunkett, E. R. Effects of dietary fat on mammary carcinogenesis by 7, 12-dimethylbenz(a)anthracene in rats. *Cancer Res.* 27:1737, 1967.
62. Garfinkel, L., Craig, L., and Seidman, H. An appraisal of left and right breast cancer. *J. Natl. Cancer Inst.* 23:617, 1959.
63. Gass, G. H., Brown, J., and Okey, A. B. Carcinogenic effects of oral diethylstilbestrol on C3H male mice with and without the mammary tumor virus. *J. Natl. Cancer Inst.* 53:1369, 1974.
64. Grattarola, R. The premenstrual endometrial pattern of women with breast cancer. *Cancer* 17:1119, 1964.
65. Grodin, J. M., Siiteri, P. K., and MacDonald, P. C. Source of

estrogen production in postmenopausal women. *J. Clin. Endocrinol. Metab.* 36:207, 1973.

66. Gross, J., Modan, B., Bertini, B., et al. Relationship between steroid excretion patterns and breast cancer incidence in Israeli women of various origins. *J. Natl. Cancer Inst.* 59:7, 1977.

67. Haagensen, C. D. *Diseases of the Breast* (2nd ed.). Philadelphia: Saunders, 1971.

68. Haagensen, C. D. The relationship of gross cystic disease of the breast and carcinoma. *Ann. Surg.* 185:375, 1977.

69. Heinonen, O. P., Shapiro, S., Tuonimen, L., et al. Reserpine use in relation to breast cancer. *Lancet* 2:675, 1974.

70. Hems, G. Epidemiological characteristics of breast cancer in middle and late age. *Br. J. Cancer* 24:226, 1970.

71. Henderson, B. E. Type B virus and human breast cancer. *Cancer* 34:1386, 1974.

72. Henderson, B. E., Gerkins, V., Rosario, I., et al. Elevated serum levels of estrogen and prolactin in daughters of patients with breast cancer. *N. Engl. J. Med.* 293:790, 1975.

73. Henderson, B. E., Powell, D., Rosario, I., et al. An epidemiologic study of breast cancer. *J. Natl. Cancer Inst.* 53:609, 1974.

74. Hennekens, C. H., Speizer, F. E., Rosner, B., et al. Hair dyes and human cancer (abstract). *Am. J. Epidemiol.* 108:240, 1978.

75. Hill, P., Wynder, E. L., Kumar, J., et al. Prolactin levels in populations at risk for breast cancer. *Cancer Res.* 36:4102, 1976.

76. Hirayama, T., and Wynder, E. L. A study of the epidemiology of cancer of the breast: II. The influence of hysterectomy. *Cancer* 15:28, 1962.

77. Hoover, R., Gray, L. W., Sr., Cole, P., et al. Menopausal estrogens and breast cancer. *N. Engl. J. Med.* 295:401, 1976.

78. Humphrey, L. J., and Swerdlow, M. The relationship of breast cancer to thyroid disease. *Cancer* 17:1170, 1964.

79. Humphrey, L. J., and Swerdlow, M. A. Large duct epithelial hyperplasia and carcinoma of the breast. *Arch. Surg.* 97:592, 1968.

80. Jablon, S., and Kato, H. Studies of mortality of A-bomb survivors: 5. Radiation dose and mortality, 1950–1970. *Radiat. Res.* 50:649, 1972.

81. Kapde, C. C., and Wolfe, J. N. Breast cancer: Relationship to thyroid supplements for hypothyroidism. *J.A.M.A.* 236:1124, 1976.

82. Kaplan, S. D., and Acheson, R. M. A single etiological hypothesis for breast cancer? *J. Chronic Dis.* 19:1221, 1966.

83. Kelsey, J. L., Holford, T. R., White, C., et al. Oral contraceptives and breast disease: An epidemiological study. *Am. J. Epidemiol.* 107:236, 1978.

84. Kewitz, H., Jesdinsky, J. H., Shroter, P. M., et al. Reserpine and breast cancer in West Germany. *Eur. J. Clin. Pharmacol.* 11:79, 1977.

85. Kinlen, L. J., Harris, R., Garrod, A., et al. Use of hair dyes by patients with breast cancer: A case-control study. *Br. Med. J.* 2:366, 1977.
86. Kirschner, M. A. The role of hormones in the etiology of human breast cancer. *Cancer* 39:2716, 1977.
87. Kodlin, D., Winger, E. E., Morgenstern, N. L., et al. Chronic mastopathy and breast cancer. A follow-up study. *Cancer* 39:2603, 1977.
88. Krook, P. M., Carlile, T., Bush, W., et al. Mammographic parenchymal patterns as a risk indicator for prevalent and incident cancer. *Cancer* 41:1093, 1978.
89. Kumaoka, S., Takatami, O., Abe, O., et al. Plasma prolactin, thyroid-stimulating hormone, follicle-stimulating hormone and luteinizing hormone in normal British and Japanese women. *Eur. J. Cancer* 12:767, 1976.
90. Land, C. E., and McGregor, D. H. Breast cancer incidence among atomic bomb survivors: Implications for radiobiologic risk at low doses. *J. Natl. Cancer Inst.* 62:17, 1979.
91. Laska, E. M., Siegel, C., Meisner, M., et al. Matched-pairs study of reserpine use and breast cancer. *Lancet* 2:296, 1975.
92. Lemon, H. M. Experimental basis for multiple primary carcinogenesis by sex hormones. *Cancer* 40:1825, 1977.
93. Lemon, H. M., Wotiz, H. H., Parsons, L., et al. Reduced estriol excretion in patients with breast cancer prior to endocrine therapy. *J.A.M.A.* 196:1128, 1966.
94. Lewison, E. F., and Lyons, J. G. Relationship between benign breast disease and cancer. *Arch. Surg.* 66:94, 1953.
95. Lilienfeld, A. M. The relationship of cancer of the female breast to artificial menopause and marital status. *Cancer* 9:927, 1956.
96. Lilienfeld, A. M., Chang, L., Thomas, D. B., et al. Rauwolfia derivatives and breast cancer. *Johns Hopkins Med. J.* 139:41, 1976.
97. Lilienfeld, A. M., Coombs, J., Bross, I. D. J., et al. Marital and reproductive experience in a community-wide epidemiological study of breast cancer. *Johns Hopkins Med. J.* 136:157, 1975.
98. Lin, T. M., Chen, K. P., and MacMahon, B. Epidemiologic characteristics of cancer of the breast in Taiwan. *Cancer* 27:1497, 1971.
99. Lipsett, M. B. Oestrogen profiles and breast cancer. *Lancet* 2:1378, 1971.
100. LiVolsi, V. A., Stadel, B. V., Kelsey, J. L., et al. Fibrocystic breast disease in oral contraceptive users: A histopathologic evaluation of epithelial atypia. *N. Engl. J. Med.* 299:381, 1978.
101. Longcope, C., and Pratt, J. H. Relationship between urine and plasma estrogen ratios. *Cancer Res.* 38:4025, 1978.
102. Lynch, H. I., and Krush, A. J. Genetic predictability in breast cancer risk. *Arch. Surg.* 103:84, 1971.
103. Mack, T. M., Henderson, B. E., Gerkins, V. R., et al. Reserpine

and breast cancer in a retirement community. *N. Engl. J. Med.* 292:1366, 1975.

104. MacKenzie, I. Breast cancer following multiple fluoroscopies. *Br. J. Cancer* 19:1, 1965.

105. Macklin, M. T. Comparison of the number of breast-cancer deaths observed in relatives of breast-cancer patients, and the number expected on the basis of mortality rates. *J. Natl. Cancer Inst.* 22:927, 1959.

106. MacMahon, B., and Austin, J. H. Association of carcinomas of the breast and corpus uteri. *Cancer* 23:275, 1969.

107. MacMahon, B., and Cole, P. The Ovarian Etiology of Human Breast Cancer. In E. Grundmann, and H. Tulinius (Eds.), *Current Problems in the Epidemiology of Cancer and Lymphomas.* New York: Springer-Verlag, 1972.

108. MacMahon, B., Cole, P., and Brown, J. Etiology of human breast cancer: A review. *J. Natl. Cancer Inst.* 50:21, 1973.

109. MacMahon, B., Cole, P., Brown, J. B., et al. Estrogen profiles of Asian and North American women. *Int. J. Cancer* 14:161, 1974.

110. MacMahon, B., Cole, P., Lin, T. M., et al. Age at first birth and breast cancer risk. *Bull. WHO* 43:209, 1970.

111. MacMahon, B., and Feinleib, M. Breast cancer in relation to nursing and menopausal history. *J. Natl. Cancer Inst.* 24:733, 1960.

112. MacMahon, B., Lin, T. M., Lowe, C. R., et al. Lactation and cancer of the breast. A summary of an international study. *Bull. WHO* 42:185, 1970.

113. McDivitt, R. W., Hutter, R. V., Foote, F. W., Jr., et al. In situ lobular carcinoma. A prospective follow-up study indicating cumulative patient risks. *J.A.M.A.* 201:96, 1967.

114. McGregor, D. H., Land, C. E., Choi, K., et al. Breast cancer incidence among atomic bomb survivors, Hiroshima and Nagasaki, 1950–1969. *J. Natl. Cancer Inst.* 59:799, 1977.

115. McManus, I. C. Predominance of left-sided breast tumours. *Lancet* 2:297, 1977.

116. Menck, H. R., Pike, M. C., Henderson, B. E., et al. Lung cancer risk among beauticians and other female workers: Brief communication. *J. Natl. Cancer Inst.* 59:1423, 1977.

117. Mendell, L., Rosenbloom, M., and Maimark, A. Are breast patterns a risk index for breast cancer? A reappraisal. *A.J.R.* 128:547, 1977.

118. Mettler, F. A., Jr., Hempelmann, L. H., Dutton, A. M., et al. Breast neoplasms in women treated with X-rays for acute postpartum mastitis. A pilot study. *J. Natl. Cancer Inst.* 43:803, 1969.

119. Miller, A. B. Role of nutrition in the etiology of breast cancer. *Cancer* 39:2704, 1977.

120. Miller, A. B., Kelly, A., Choi, N. W., et al. A study of diet and breast cancer. *Am. J. Epidemiol.* 107:499, 1978.

121. Modan, B., Barell, V., Lubin, F., et al. Dietary factors and cancer in Israel. *Cancer Res.* 35:3503, 1975.
122. Monson, R. R., Yen, S., MacMahon, B., et al. Chronic mastitis and carcinoma of the breast. *Lancet* 2:224, 1976.
123. Muhlbock, O., and Boot, L. M. The mode of action of ovarian hormones in the induction of mammary cancer in mice. *Biochem. Pharmacol.* 16:627, 1967.
124. Mustacchi, P., and Greenspan, F. Thyroid supplementation for hypothyroidism: An iatrogenic cause of breast cancer? *J.A.M.A.* 237:1446, 1977.
125. Mydren, J. A., and Hiltz, J. E. Breast cancer following multiple fluoroscopies during artificial pneumothorax treatment of pulmonary tuberculosis. *Can. Med. Assoc. J.* 100:1032, 1969.
126. National Cancer Institute Ad Hoc Working Groups on Mammography Screening for Breast Cancer. First Reports and a Summary Report of Their Joint Findings and Recommendations (DHEW Publication No. NIH 77-1400). Washington, D. C.: U.S. Government Printing Office, March, 1977.
127. O'Fallon, W. M., Labarthe, D. R., and Kurland, L. T. Rauwolfia derivatives and breast cancer. A case-control study in Olmstead County, Minnesota. *Lancet* 2:292, 1975.
128. Ory, H., Cole, P., MacMahon, B., et al. Oral contraceptives and reduced risk of benign breast diseases. *N. Engl. J. Med.* 294:419, 1976.
129. Paffenbarger, R. S., Fasal, E., Simmons, M. E., et al. Cancer risk as related to use of oral contraceptives during fertile years. *Cancer* 39(Suppl.):1887, 1977.
130. Page, B. L., Vander Zwaag, R., Rogers, L. W., et al. Relation between component parts of fibrocystic disease complex and breast cancer. *J. Natl. Cancer Inst.* 61:1055, 1978.
131. Peyster, R. G., Kalisher, L., and Cole, P. Mammographic parenchymal patterns and the prevalence of breast cancer. *Radiology* 125:387, 1977.
132. Phillips, R. L. Role of life-style and dietary habits in risk of cancer among Seventh-Day Adventists. *Cancer Res.* 35:3513, 1975.
133. Pike, M. C., Casagrande, J. T., Brown, J. B., et al. Comparison of urinary and plasma hormone levels in daughters of breast cancer patients and controls. *J. Natl. Cancer Inst.* 59:1351, 1977.
134. Poel, W. E. Progesterone enhancement of mammary development as a causal model of co-carcinogenesis. *Br. J. Cancer* 22:867, 1968.
135. Potter, J. F., Slimbaugh, W. P., Woodward, S. C. Can breast carcinoma be anticipated? A follow-up of benign breast biopsies. *Ann. Surg.* 167:829, 1968.
136. Rader, M. D., Flickinger, D. L., de Villa, G. U., Jr., et al. Plasma estrogens in postmenopausal women, *Am. J. Obstet. Gynecol.* 116:1069, 1973.

137. Ravnihar, B., MacMahon, B., and Lindtner, J. Epidemiologic features of breast cancer in Slovenia, 1965–1967. *Eur. J. Cancer* 7:295, 1971.

138. Reemer, R. R., Hoover, R., Fraumeni, J. F., Jr., et al. Second primary neoplasms following ovarian cancer. *J. Natl. Cancer Inst.* 61:1195, 1978.

139. Rideout, D. F., and Poon, P. Y. Patterns of breast parenchyma in mammography. *J. Can. Assoc. Radiol.* 28:257, 1977.

140. Robbins, G. F., and Berg, J. W. Bilateral primary breast cancers: A prospective clinicopathological study. *Cancer* 17:1501, 1964.

141. Royal College of General Practitioners. *Oral Contraceptives and Health.* New York: Pitman, 1974.

142. Royal College of General Practitioners. Oral contraceptive study: Effect on hypertension and benign breast disease of progestagen component in combined oral contraceptives. *Lancet* 1:624, 1977.

143. Rudali, G., Apiou, F., and Muel, B. Mammary cancer produced in mice with oestriol. *Eur. J. Cancer* 2:39, 1975.

144. Salber, E. J., Trichopoulos, D., and MacMahon, B. Lactation and reproductive histories of breast cancer patients in Boston 1965–1966. *J. Natl. Cancer Inst.* 43:1013, 1969.

145. Sartwell, P. E., Arthes, F. G., and Tonascia, J. A. Epidemiology of benign breast lesions: Lack of associations with oral contraceptive use. *N. Engl. J. Med.* 288:551, 1973.

146. Sartwell, P. E., Arthes, F. G., and Tonascia, J. A. Exogenous hormones, reproductive history, and breast cancer. *J. Natl. Cancer Inst.* 59:1589, 1977.

147. Sasaki, G. H., and Leung, B. S. On the mechanism of action of hormone action in 7,12-dimethylbenz(a)anthracene-induced mammary tumor. *Cancer* 35:645, 1975.

148. Schindler, A. E., Ebert, A., and Friedrich, E. Conversion of androstenedione to estrone by human fat tissue. *J. Clin. Endocrinol. Metab.* 35:627, 1972.

149. Schoenberg, B. S. Multiple Primary Neoplasms. In J. F. Fraumeni, Jr. (Ed.), *Persons at High Risk of Cancer.* New York: Academic, 1975.

150. Schoenberg, B. S. *Multiple Primary Malignant Neoplasms: The Connecticut Experience, 1935–1964.* New York: Springer-Verlag, 1977.

151. Schottenfeld, D., and Berg, J. Incidence of multiple primary cancers: IV. Cancers of the female breast and genital organs. *J. Natl. Cancer Inst.* 46:161, 1971.

152. Schottenfeld, D., and Berg, J. Epidemiology of Multiple Primary Cancers. In D. Schottenfeld (Ed.), *Cancer Epidemiology and Prevention. Current Concepts.* Springfield, Ill.: Thomas, 1975.

153. Searle, C. E., Harnden, D. G., Venitt, S., et al. Carcinogenicity and mutagenicity tests of some hair colourants and constituents. *Nature* 255:506, 1975.

154. SEER Program. Cancer Incidence and Mortality in the United

States 1973–1976. (Edited by J. L. Young, Jr., A. J. Asire, and E. S. Pollack. DHEW Publication No. NIH 78-1837.) Bethesda, Md., 1978.

155. Shafer, N., and Shafer, R. W. Potential of carcinogenic effects of hair dyes. *N.Y. State J. Med.* 76:394, 1976.

156. Shapiro, S. Evidence on screening for breast cancer from a randomized trial. *Cancer* 39:2772, 1977.

157. Sherman, B. M., and Korenman, S. G. Inadequate corpus luteum function: A pathophysiological interpretation of human breast cancer epidemiology. *Cancer* 33:1306, 1974.

158. Shore, R. E., Hempelmann, L. H., Kowaluk, E., et al. Breast neoplasms in women treated with x-rays for acute postpartum mastitis. *J. Natl. Cancer Inst.* 59:813, 1977.

159. Shore, R. E., Pasternack, B. S., Thiessen, E. U., et al. A case-control study of hair dye use and breast cancer. *J. Natl. Cancer Inst.* 62:277, 1979.

160. Siiteri, P. K., Schwarz, B. E., and MacDonald, P. C. Estrogen receptors and the estrone hypothesis in relation to endometrial and breast cancer. *Gynecol. Oncol.* 2:228, 1974.

161. Sloss, P. T., Bennett, W. A., and Clagett, O. T. Incidence in normal breasts of features associated with chronic cystic mastitis. *Am. J. Pathol.* 33:1181, 1957.

162. Staszewski, J. Age at menarche and breast cancer. *J. Natl. Cancer Inst.* 47:935, 1971.

163. Stavraky, K., and Emmons, S. Breast cancer in premenopausal and postmenopausal women. *J. Natl. Cancer Inst.* 53:647, 1974.

164. Stocks, P. Breast cancer anomalies. *Br. J. Cancer* 24:633, 1970.

165. Swain, M. C., Bulbrook, R. D., and Hayward, J. L. Ovulatory failure in a normal population and in patients with breast cancer. *J. Obstet. Gynecol. Br. Commonw.* 81:640, 1974.

166. Thein-Hlang, Thein-Maung-Myint. Risk factors of breast cancer in Burma. *Int. J. Cancer* 21:432, 1978.

167. Tokuhata, G. K. Morbidity and mortality among offspring of breast cancer mothers. *Am. J. Epidemiol.* 89:139, 1969.

168. Trichopoulos, D., MacMahon, B., and Cole, P. Menopause and breast cancer risk. *J. Natl. Cancer Inst.* 48:605, 1972.

169. Tulinius, H., Day, N. E., Johannesson, G., et al. Reproductive factors and risk for breast cancer in Iceland. *Int. J. Cancer* 21:724, 1978.

170. Vessey, M. P., Doll, R., and Jones, K. Oral contraceptives and breast cancer. *Lancet* 1:941, 1975.

171. Vessey, M. P., Doll, R., Peto, R., et al. A long-term follow-up study of women using different methods of contraception—an interim report. *J. Biosoc. Sci.* 8:373, 1976.

172. Vessey, M. P., Doll, R., and Sutton, P. M. Oral contraceptives and breast neoplasia: A retrospective study. *Br. Med. J.* 3:719, 1972.

173. Vongtoma, V., Kurohara, S. S., Badib, A. O., et al. Second primary cancers of endometrial carcinoma. *Cancer* 26:842, 1970.

174. Wallace, R. B., Sherman, B. M., Bean, J. A., et al. Thyroid hormone use in patients with breast cancer. Absence of an association. *J.A.M.A.* 239:948, 1978.
175. Wallach, S., and Henneman, P. H. Prolonged estrogen therapy in postmenopausal women. *J.A.M.A.* 171:1637, 1959.
176. Walrath, J. Cancer incidence amongst cosmetologists. Yale University, Ph.D. Thesis, 1977.
177. Wanebo, C. K., Johnson, K. G., Sato, K., et al. Breast cancer after exposure to the atomic bombings of Hiroshima and Nagasaki. *N. Engl. J. Med.* 279:667, 1968.
178. Wilkinson, E., Clopton, C., Gordonson, J., et al. Mammographic parenchymal pattern and the risk of breast cancer. *J. Natl. Cancer Inst.* 59:1397, 1977.
179. Wilson, R. A. The roles of estrogen and progesterone in breast and genital cancer. *J.A.M.A.* 182:327, 1962.
180. Wolfe, J. N. A study of breast parenchyma by mammography in the normal woman and those with benign and malignant disease. *Radiology* 89:201, 1967.
181. Wolfe, J. N. Breast parenchymal patterns and their changes with age. *Radiology* 121:545, 1976.
182. Wolfe, J. N. Breast patterns as an index of risk for developing breast cancer. *A.J.R.* 126:1130, 1976.
183. Wolfe, J. N. Risk for breast cancer development determined by mammographic parenchymal pattern. *Cancer* 37:2486, 1976.
184. Wynder, E. L., Bross, J. J., and Hirayama, T. A study of the epidemiology of cancer of the breast. *Cancer* 13:559, 1960.
185. Wynder, E. L., Hyams, L., and Shijematsu, T. Correlation of international cancer death rates. *Cancer* 20:113, 1967.
186. Yuasa, S., and MacMahon, B. Lactation and reproductive histories of breast cancer patients in Tokyo, Japan. *Bull. WHO* 42:195, 1970.
187. Zdeb, M. S. The probability of developing cancer. *Am. J. Epidemiol.* 106:6, 1977.
188. Zumoff, B., Fishman, J., Bradlow, H. J., et al. Hormone profiles in hormone dependent cancer. *Cancer Res.* 35:3365, 1975.

Robert T. Osteen
Aziza Soliman-Fam

2. Surgical Anatomy of the Breast

The breast is a compound alveolar gland that develops from multiple invaginations of the surface ectodermal cells of the embryo at the site of the future nipple [1]. Each of these invaginations develops into a lobe of the future mammary gland and is connected to the nipple by a single excretory duct. At birth, the male and female breast are similar in structure and consist of 15 to 20 ducts radiating from the nipple. While the male gland remains undeveloped, the female breast starts to develop 2 to 3 years prior to puberty in response to complex hormonal control. The primary ducts branch and rebranch to form a conical mass as the nipple and areola enlarge. The breast then gradually assumes its rounded, mature feminine shape.

Gross Anatomy of the Mature Breast

The superficial fascia of the anterior thoracoabdominal wall consists of a superficial fatty layer and a deeper membranous layer. The mammary gland grows into this superficial fatty layer and acquires a covering of fat. A layer of membranous fascia immediately under the skin may be demonstrated radiographically. Posterior to the glandular tissue is a potential space—the retromammary space—between the deep membranous fascia and the dense pectoral fascia. Small branches of the thoracoacromial artery traverse this space to perforate the pectoralis major muscle and supply the posterior surface of the mammary gland. Large lymphatic ducts originate from the posterior surface of the gland, cross the retromammary space, and pierce the pectoral fascia and pectoralis major muscle. These lymphatics pass through the intercostal spaces to join the internal mammary lymph trunks or pass laterally to join the axillary nodes.

By injecting lactiferous ducts with methylene blue, Hicken [13] demonstrated the relationship of breast tissue to the chest wall. Figure 2–1 shows that ducts and glandular tissue may be widely distributed over the chest wall, with extension of breast tissue into the axillary recess in 95 percent of cases. Breast tissue may extend toward the epigastrium in 15 percent of cases,

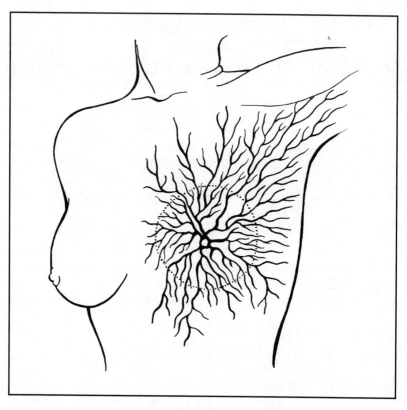

Figure 2–1. A composite drawing of the extent of lactiferous ducts over the chest wall. (From W. H. Hollinshead, *Anatomy for Surgeons: The Thorax, Abdomen, and Pelvis* [2nd ed.]. New York: Harper & Row, 1971. P. 12; after N. F. Hicken, *Arch. Surg.* 40:6, 1940.)

across the midline in 0.5 percent, and laterally to the posterior axillary line in 2 percent. Because of this wide distribution of breast tissue, the anatomic limits of a mastectomy are the clavicle, the midline, the rectus sheath, and the latissimus dorsi muscle. Even with these boundaries, some mastectomies are probably incomplete.

During development, each of the original 15 to 20 primary ducts forms a lobe, which is then subdivided into lobules. These lobules differ in size and number and consist of secretory ducts and alveoli that drain into the main excretory duct of the lobe. The lobes are separated from each other by dense, interlobular connective tissue, while the lobules are separated by a looser, more cellular, connective tissue that allows for hypertrophy during pregnancy. After several pregnancies, the breast often becomes less homogeneous to palpation, and distinct lobular masses of normal breast tissue may be confused with neoplasms.

The breast's dense, interlobular network of connective tissue was first described by Cooper [5]. Fibrous projections from the posterior aspect of the breast cross the retromammary space to the pectoral fascia, and breast tissue may reach as far as the pectoralis major muscle. These projections have provided one anatomic rationale for resection of the pectoralis major muscle in a radical mastectomy. The fibrous network also forms archlike projections from the outer surface of the glandular tissue to the superficial fascia located under the skin. Cooper's ligaments suspend the breast from overlying skin. The amount of elastic tissue in the skin of the breast varies among different individuals and different races, and Cooper's ligaments are not the only element of support to the breast. The elastic fibers of the skin may be more important than the suspensory ligaments in preserving the shape of the breast.

In 1892, Stiles [18] showed that small projections of breast parenchyma may follow Cooper's ligaments to the deep layers of the skin. However, the overlying skin is not part of the breast, and invasion of the skin by breast cancer is invasion of an adjacent organ, implying a poorer prognosis than is the case when the tumor is confined to the tissue of origin. The lymphatics from the superficial portions of the breast communicate with the skin lymphatics by way of Cooper's ligaments. Invasion of the dermal lymphatics is a manifestation of advanced breast cancer. When the dermal lymphatics are obstructed by cancer, the skin becomes edematous, taking on the so-called *peau d'or-ange* appearance.

Histology of the Resting Breast Parenchyma

The basic unit of the breast is a lobule composed of ducts and alveoli. Both are secretory in nature and are lined by cuboidal or low columnar epithelium. Early in the menstrual cycle these ducts have no lumina and are solid cords of epithelial cells. Prior to the end of the cycle, ductal cells become columnar, and a small lumen is evident. Periductal connective tissue becomes more vascular, causing the premenstrual breast engorgement that some women experience. The epithelial cells lining the secretory ducts and alveoli are situated superior to a basolamina. A myoepithelial network is responsible for the ejection of milk from the secretory cells into the lumen of the alveolar ducts. The alveolar ducts, ultimately draining into a single excretory duct, course beneath the skin of the areola and form dilations called milk sinuses. About 15 to 20 ducts converge toward the nipple, where they open separately. In the substance of the nipple, the excretory ducts terminate in ampullae at the tip of the nipple. The ampullae are lined with stratified squamous epithelium. Smooth, longitudinal, and circular muscle sur-rounds the excretory ducts in the substance of the nipple.

The Nipple and Areola

The skin of the nipple and areola is devoid of fat. It contains a layer of circumferential smooth muscle at its base, responsible for tactile nipple erection. Color is attributed to dermal papillae growing into the skin and bringing blood close to the surface [4]. The areola possesses multiple, large sweat glands, called the glands of Montgomery. Coarse hairs and sebaceous glands are seen at the periphery of the areola.

Axillary Fascia

The deep fascia over the pectoralis major muscle is dense and has septae between the muscle bundles. It is attached superiorly to the clavicle, medially to the sternum, and laterally to a thin layer of fascia enclosing the pectoralis minor muscle (Fig. 2–2).

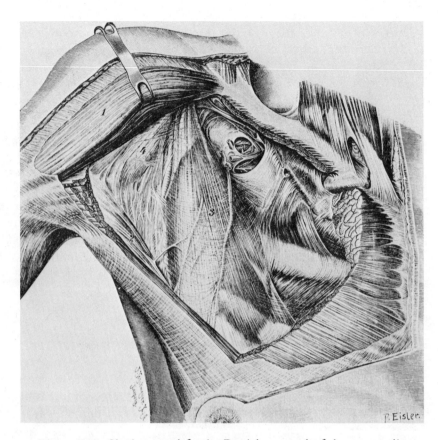

Figure 2–2. Clavipectoral fascia. Partial removal of the pectoralis major muscle exposes the pectoral minor muscle (*3*), with the clavipectoral fascia medially and the axillary fascia laterally (*4*). (From P. Eisler, *Handbuch der Anatomie des Menschen.* Jena: Gustav Fischer, 1912.)

The lateral extent of the deep fascia forms the costocoracoid membrane between the medial border of the pectoralis minor and the first rib. Superiorly, the fascia encloses the subclavius muscle and attaches to the undersurface of the clavicle. From the lateral border of the pectoralis minor muscle, it crosses the axilla into the proximal forearm as a thick sheet of connective tissue containing fat, lymph vessels, and the lymph nodes, that are removed en masse during a radical mastectomy. The axillary tail of the breast pierces the axillary fascia and is positioned directly over the serratus anterior muscle. Contraction of the pectoral muscles tightens the axillary fascia and may inhibit the palpation of axillary lymph nodes and the tail of the breast. If the elbow is supported and the arm slightly abducted by the examiner, the pectoral muscles are relaxed, facilitating examination of the axilla.

Blood Supply of the Breast

Arteries

The mammary gland is supplied by medial branches from the internal thoracic (internal mammary) artery, lateral branches from the axillary artery, and smaller inferior branches from the intercostal arteries (Fig. 2–3). The posterior aspect of the breast is supplied by branches of the thoracoacromial artery, which perforate the pectoralis major muscle.

Medial Arteries. The internal thoracic branch of the subclavian artery sends anterior and medial perforating branches into the first four intercostal spaces. These vessels supply the internal intercostal muscles, the external intercostal membrane, and the sternal fibers of the pectoralis major muscle. Glandular branches to the breast usually arise from the first two branches of the internal thoracic artery. These branches pass obliquely downward toward the areola and share several anastomotic arcades with the lateral arteries before reaching the areola.

Lateral Arteries. The lateral arteries are branches of the axillary artery by way of the lateral thoracic or subscapular arteries. The subscapular artery frequently supplies the lower lateral quadrant of the mammary gland.

Inferior Arteries. The inferior arteries are constant intercostal branches that pierce the fifth and sometimes the sixth intercostal

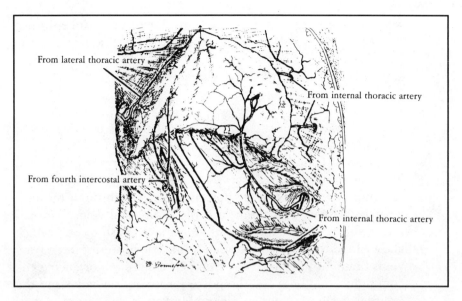

Figure 2–3. Arterial supply of the breast. (From M. Salmon, *Ann. Anat. Path.* 16:477, 1939.)

spaces. There are two groups of inferior or posterior arteries: the medial branches from the internal thoracic artery and the lateral branches from the intercostal artery. The inferior arteries may also contribute to the circumareolar vascular ring.

Veins

Blood flow through the superficial veins tends to be directed medially toward the internal thoracic vein. The deeper veins are directed laterally toward two or three large veins that drain into the axillary vein. Inferiorly, one or two small veins may accompany the inferior or posterior arteries through the fifth intercostal space and drain into the intercostal veins. The anterior and posterior intercostal veins have anastomoses, which allow blood to flow in either direction. The posterior intercostal veins drain into the azygos system. Of clinical importance is the communication between the posterior intercostal veins and the internal vertebral venous plexus by way of the intervertebral foramina. Described by Batson [3], these communicating veins are devoid of valves, so malignant emboli from the breast may metastasize into the vertebrae, the pleura, or any of the osseous structures associated with the vertebral plexus from the pelvis and the upper end of the femur to the shoulder girdle and the skull.

Nerves of the Breast

Stimulation of the nipple induces reflex secretion of prolactin and oxytocin for lactation. For this function there is a rich supply of sensory endings, particularly in the nipple and skin. The glandular tissue is less well innervated.

Supraclavicular nerves innervate only the skin of the breast. Other contributions to innervation of the skin and the entire supply of the glandular tissue are from the second through the seventh intercostal nerves. The anterior cutaneous branches of these intercostal nerves accompany the perforating branches of the internal thoracic artery. The axillary process of the breast is supplied by the intercostal brachial nerve and the third and fourth lateral cutaneous nerves.

According to Craig and Sykes [6], the nipple and the areola are always supplied from the depth of the breast. Edwards [9] has described a single special nerve, a branch of the fourth lateral cutaneous nerve, which passes directly through the breast to the nipple.

Lymphatic Drainage of the Breast

In the 18th century, Cruikshank [7] and Mascagni [15] used mercury injection of cadavers to identify the two main routes of lymphatic flow from the breast: an external (or lateral) outflow, which accompanies the lateral thoracic blood vessels to the axilla, and an internal (or medial) outflow, which follows the anterior perforating branches of the internal thoracic blood vessels and drains into the internal thoracic lymphatic chain (Fig. 2–4). A century later, Sappey [17] described the superficial lymphatics of the anterior thoracoabdominal wall. The superficial lymphatics above the umbilicus usually drain into the axillary nodes. The deeper lymphatics of the breast along the excretory ducts join the subareolar lymphatic plexus. Large lymph trunks arise from the medial and lateral borders of this plexus and either pass laterally to the axilla or medially to the internal thoracic chain. Turner-Warwick [19] and others [11, 14] supplemented the anatomic studies with information derived from intravital injection of dye and radioactive colloidal gold. Results confirmed the previous view that lymphatics follow blood vessels and, in addition, that the lymphatic drainage is approximately proportionate to the blood supply. Therefore, most (75%) of the lymphatic drainage from the breast is into the axillary nodes. Approximately 25 percent of the lymph flow is to the parasternal nodes, with the posterior intercostal nodes only receiving about 2 percent.

Classification of the Axillary Nodes

The axillary nodes are commonly classified into six groups, as shown in Figure 2–5.

External Mammary Nodes. The external mammary nodes consist of small nodes along the course of the lateral thoracic blood vessels, beneath the lateral border of the pectoralis major muscle. They are loosely attached to the fascia of the serratus anterior muscle. Despite their proximity to the breast, the external mammary nodes have been found to be involved in only 7.2 percent of cases of breast carcinoma with metastases in the axillary nodes. Therefore, procedures that sample only these

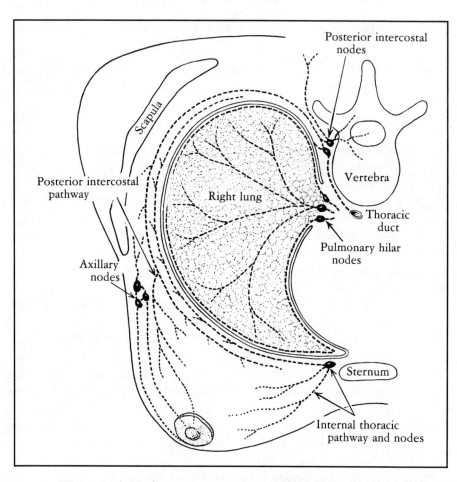

Figure 2–4. Mediastinal connections of lymphatics from the breast. (From E. Edwards, Surgical Anatomy of the Breast. In R. M. Goldwyn (Ed.), *Plastic and Reconstructive Surgery of the Breast.* Boston: Little, Brown, 1976. P. 48; after C. H. Leaf, *Cancer of the Breast: Clinically Considered.* London: Constable & Co., 1912.)

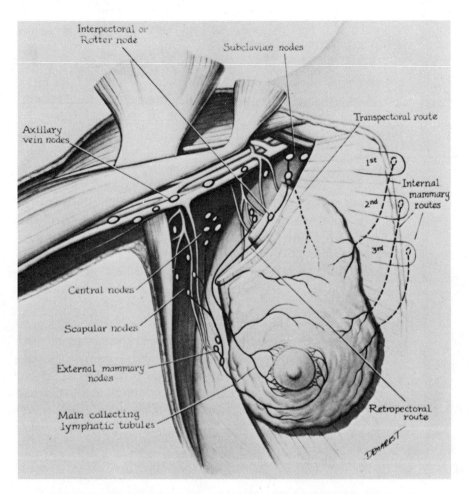

Figure 2–5. Lymphatics and lymph node groups: pectoral nodes, interpectoral nodes, central nodes, axillary vein nodes, nodes draining the arm, apical or subclavicular nodes, supraclavicular nodes, lymph trunks draining into the internal thoracic trunks. (From C. D. Haagensen, *Disease of the Breast* [2nd ed.]. Philadelphia: Saunders, 1971. P. 33.)

lymph nodes for prognosis of breast cancer may miss a substantial number of metastases.

Subscapular Nodes. The subscapular nodes, a group of five or six nodes, are found along the course of the subscapular blood vessels at the posterior axillary fold. They lie in close proximity to the thoracodorsal nerve, which can be damaged during dissection of these nodes.

Interpectoral Nodes (Rotter's Nodes). Lymphatic trunks from the posterior aspect of the breast traverse the retromammary space to reach the interpectoral nodes, which are located between the pectoralis major and minor muscles, along the course of the pectoral branches of the thoracoacromial blood vessels. In 1899, Rotter [16] found that in 33 percent of surgically removed breasts the interpectoral nodes were affected by malignancy. In more modern series, probably dealing with less extensive disease, the incidence of metastases to the interpectoral nodes is much lower.

Central Nodes. The central nodes are the largest and most easily palpated nodes in the axilla. They lie superficially beneath the axillary skin and are the most common group of nodes involved with metastases from carcinoma of the breast.

Axillary Vein Nodes. The axillary vein lymph nodes are located anterior and caudad to the lateral part of the vein. They are not easily palpated because they are covered by the thick tendon of the pectoralis major muscle. Lymphatics from the posterior surface of the breast ascend upward and laterally to enter the axillary vein nodes. If these lymphatics are interrupted by meticulously stripping the axillary vein of its adventitia during a radical mastectomy, a swollen arm may result.

Subclavicular Nodes (Apical Nodes). The subclavicular nodes are the continuation of the axillary vein nodes and are medial to the tendon of the pectoralis minor muscle at the anatomic apex of the axilla. Lymphatics from the posterior surface of the breast may traverse the retromammary space, enter the pectoralis major muscle, and ascend medially and upward to the subclavicular nodes. These lymphatics also may take the lateral course to the retromammary space at the border of the pectoralis major muscle, pass between the pectoralis major and minor muscles, and follow the pectoral branches of the thoracoacromial artery to the subclavicular nodes. Lymphatics from the axillary vein group as well as from the central nodes may also reach the subclavicular nodes. Because of their location posterior to the clavipectoral fascia (costocoracoid membrane), the apical lymph nodes can be reached most conveniently by removal or division of the pectoralis major and minor muscles. Involvement of the apical nodes by metastases is a manifestation of advanced carcinoma of the breast and indicates a poor prognosis. The standard radical mastectomy in which pectoral muscles are removed differs from the "modified" radical mastectomy in that the apical nodes are more accessible and more readily removed in the former operation. Auchincloss [2] has questioned the therapeutic efficacy of removing the apical nodes pointing out that of 204 patients subjected to radical mastectomy, only four might have benefited from removal of the apical nodes. The other 200 either had no involvement of the apical nodes or died of systemic metastases.

Supraclavicular Nodes
The supraclavicular nodes form part of the deep lymphatic system in the neck immediately above the clavicle. The lymphatics of the head and neck and the supraclavicular nodes ultimately drain into the inferior cervical nodes located deep to the clavicular head of the sternocleidomastoid muscle adjacent to the lower part of the internal jugular vein. Involvement of the supraclavicular nodes by metastatic carcinoma of the breast is an indication of systemic disease.

Internal Mammary Lymphatics
Two or three lymphatic trunks course on either side of the sternum. They begin caudally, posterior to the sixth intercostal space, by the union of smaller lymphatics from the anterior part of the diaphragm, the anterior superior surfaces of the liver, the rectus sheath, and the rectus abdominis muscle. They extend craniad, paralleling the internal thoracic vessels, and are interrupted along their course by small lymph nodes, one in each of the upper three intercostal spaces and a fourth opposite the sixth intercostal space. The lymphatic trunks and lymph nodes are ensheathed between two layers of fascia posterior to which is the parietal pleura. About half of the time, the right and left lymphatic trunks are interconnected at the level of the first intercostal space.

Handley and Thackray [12] biopsied lymph nodes from the

upper three intercostal spaces of 150 patients with clinically operable breast carcinoma. These studies first documented that invasion of the internal mammary chain may occur in patients who, by all other criteria, have curable breast cancer. Of the 150 patients, 33 percent had metastases to the internal mammary nodes at the time of operation. Interestingly, in only eight cases were the internal mammary nodes involved alone. Handley and Thackray's data are supported by more recent observations that most instances of internal mammary node involvement by carcinoma of the breast are accompanied by axillary node involvement [8, 20]. In Handley and Thackray's series, when the primary involvement was in the inner half of the breast and the axillary nodes were invaded, approximately 66 percent of the cases had internal mammary node involvement as well. In general, the greater the degree of axillary node involvement, the more likely that internal mammary disease will be present.

Lymphatic Metastases from Carcinoma of the Breast

The rationale for the en bloc resection of the breast, pectoralis muscles, and axillary contents is the theory that the most common spread of breast malignancy is by way of tumor emboli to regional lymph nodes and that those lymph nodes provide a relatively effective barrier against further spread. Although this theory may have some validity, it is probably much too simplistic. Lymph nodes do not appear to be a particularly effective barrier against the spread of tumor cells [10]. A variety of other factors, including immunologic competence, probably exert an influence on the successful implantation and growth of circulating tumor cells. The detection of metastatic breast cancer in regional lymph nodes is important. The degree of regional node involvement is related to the probability of systemic disease. Furthermore, the anatomic distribution of lymph node involvement may be related to the pattern of metastases. If the efferent flow of lymph is blocked by a malignant growth, retrograde flow of tumor emboli can occur. Blockage of internal mammary flow may lead to retrograde flow of tumor emboli along lymphatics accompanying the superior epigastric vessels to the rectus sheath and falciform ligament, and from there may pass directly to the hepatic parenchyma. This mechanism would be exclusive of blood-borne metastases to the liver.

References

1. Arey, L. B. *Developmental Anatomy: A Textbook and Laboratory Manual of Embryology* (7th ed.). Philadelphia: Saunders, 1965.
2. Auchincloss, H. Significance of location and number of axillary metastases in carcinoma of the breast: A justification for a conservative operation. *Ann. Surg.* 158:37, 1963.
3. Batson, O. V. The vertebral vein system. *A.J.R.* 78:195, 1957.
4. Bloom, W., and Fawcett, D. W. *A Textbook of Histology* (10th ed.). Philadelphia: Saunders, 1975.
5. Cooper, A. P. *The Anatomy and Diseases of the Breast.* Philadelphia: Lea & Blanchard, 1845.
6. Craig, R. D., and Sykes, P. A. Nipple sensitivity following reduction mammaplasty. *Br. J. Plast. Surg.* 23:165, 1970.
7. Cruikshank, W. *The Anatomy of the Absorbing Vessels of the Human Body.* London: G. Nichol, 1790.
8. Donegan, W. L. The influence of untreated internal mammary metastases upon the course of mammary cancer. *Cancer* 39:533, 1977.
9. Edwards, E. Surgical Anatomy of the Breast. In R. M. Goldwyn (Ed.), *Plastic and Reconstructive Surgery of the Breast.* Boston: Little, Brown, 1976.
10. Fisher, B., and Fisher, E. R. Transmigration of the lymph nodes by tumor cells. *Science* 152:1397, 1966.
11. Haagensen, C. D., Feind, C. R., Herter, F. P., Slanetz, C. A., Jr., and Weinberg, J. A. *The Lymphatics in Cancer.* Philadelphia: Saunders, 1972.
12. Handley, R. S., and Thackray, A. C. Invasion of internal mammary lymph nodes in carcinoma of the breast. *Br. Med. J.* 1:61, 1954.
13. Hicken, N. F. Mastectomy: A clinical pathologic study demonstrating why most mastectomies result in incomplete removal of the mammary gland. *Arch. Surg.* 40:6, 1940.
14. Hultborn, K. A., Larsson, L. G., and Ragnhult, I. Lymph drainage from the breast to the axillary and parasternal lymph nodes, studied with the aid of colloidal Au[198]. *Acta Radiol.* 43:52, 1955.
15. Mascagni, P. *Vasorum Lymphaticorum Corporis Humani Historia et Ichonographia.* Senis, Italy: P. Carli, 1787.
16. Rotter, J. Zür tophographie des mammocarcinoms. *Arch. F. Klin. Chir.* 58:346, 1899.
17. Sappey, P. C. *Description et Ichonographia des Vaisseaux Lymphatiques.* Paris: Delahaye, 1885.
18. Stiles, H. J. Contributions to the surgical anatomy of the breast. *Edinburgh Med. J.* 37:1099, 1892.
19. Turner-Warwick, R. T. The lymphatics of the breast. *Br. J. Surg.* 46:574, 1959.
20. Valagussa, P., Bonadonna, G., and Veronesi, U. Patterns of relapse and survival following radical mastectomy. *Cancer* 41:1170, 1978.

Richard E. Wilson

3. History and Physical Diagnosis of Breast Carcinoma

The most critical factor in the diagnosis of breast cancer is the physician's judgment in selecting patients for biopsy. All criteria for diagnosis, whether based on history, physical examination, x-ray examination, or laboratory tests, pose the ultimate question of whether or not a specific site within the breast requires a histologic diagnosis. The advances that have been made in earlier diagnosis and the selection of patients for treatment have served to identify more favorable stages of malignancy.

The History

In cases of suspected breast carcinoma, an adequate patient history consists of a description of the mass or local lesion within the breast, the presence or absence of pain or discharge from the nipple, alteration of breast or nipple contour, a survey of constitutional symptoms, and basic information about the patient and her genetic history. Certain features may not appear to be significant in a given patient, but for epidemiologic studies and for the full picture of any woman with breast cancer, it is important to solicit data in all of these categories.

Each patient will describe the mass or local lesion differently. Some will call it "a thickening," and others will refer to "a lump," "a knot," or "a growth." It is necessary to describe the patient's complaint according to her own description and to ascertain whether the patient or a physician first noted the mass. Knowledge of the location by quadrant in the breast and the presence or absence of any overlying skin changes is particularly valuable. How long the mass has been present and whether or not it has changed with the menstrual cycle can be important in the overall decision as to malignancy for a specific lesion. The size and shape of the mass are of much less consequence, but, regardless of size, shape, length of time present, or variability with menstrual cycles, the presence of a persistent area of abnormality within the breast requires accurate definition and probable biopsy. Additional points in the history concerning any breast

49

lesion should include a record of past diagnostic studies, for example, previous x-rays, biopsies, or aspirations, and any previous treatment for the lesion.

The breast undergoes a daily alteration in response to hormonal patterns during the menstrual life of the female. These changes may be associated with pain, swelling, and tenderness. Pain, likewise, is a common complaint in many breast cancers, and the pain may not necessarily be located at the site of the disease. Thus, the presence or absence of pain is not an important criterion in the diagnosis of breast cancer. More importantly, fibrocystic disease frequently coexists with malignancy, and pain in an area of sclerosing adenosis or cystic hyperplasia may occur with a carcinoma growing within adjacent dysplastic tissue. It is therefore important to obtain a history of pain, but the pain history will not necessarily be related to the lesion in question. Tenderness or swelling in the breast is often hormonally related and may or may not be related to the lesion. Most malignancies do not change their configuration with a menstrual cycle, but inflammatory tissue adjacent to breast cancer may make it seem as though changes are occurring with monthly cycles even though the malignancy remains unchanged. Therefore, no statement about the presence or absence of pain or of cyclical changes in a mass can assure the physician that a cancer is not present.

Nipple discharge may be bloody or nonbloody. The nonbloody discharges may be clear, white, or green-tinged. These discharges are almost all certainly benign. On the other hand, approximately 1 out of 10 patients with a bloody discharge has breast cancer. Clear, nonbloody discharge is usually related to some type of pituitary or hormonal imbalance, while milky or greenish discharges are related to ductal disease. It is important to question whether a discharge is present unilaterally and how long it has been present. Likewise, the relationship of nipple discharge to menstrual cycles can be of value in its assessment.

Bloody discharges require an explanation and frequently require a biopsy. Pressure on a quadrant of the breast to express the discharge will help identify the proper location for biopsy. Most bloody discharges are due to papillomas, which are benign and present close to the nipple. Usually the identification of a papilloma at operation is sufficient to negate the need for extensive biopsy. Occasionally, x-ray studies of the involved duct can identify the papilloma, but this still does not rule out the need for histologic confirmation. Nonbloody discharge does not require histologic confirmation unless repeated infection, pain, or an associated mass accompanies the discharge. Cytologic evaluation of the discharge may be of value, but a negative cytologic diagnosis with bloody discharge does not rule out malignancy.

History relating to the menarche, menstrual cycle, birth of any children, and breast-feeding is important. Any prior surgery and medication, however insignificant, should be recorded. The family history is a critical factor in the diagnosis of breast cancer and should be obtained at the patient's first visit, even if the lesion does not appear to require biopsy. The patient's genetic relationship to female relatives with breast cancer, their age at diagnosis, and the outcome of the disease are all factors that should be recorded. Other malignancy in family members should be noted, but it may not be of any importance in determining the risk factor for that patient.

The presence of weight loss, anorexia, and fever are poor prognostic signs. A cough or shortness of breath, a history of anemia, and the presence of bone pain are also critical considerations. Timing of previous chest x-rays, blood tests, and any additional diagnostic procedures should be recorded.

Physical Examination

From the standpoint of the surgeon, the physical examination is of vital importance. Regardless of the history or laboratory findings, the presence of a palpable, dominant, and persistent mass lesion is the primary indication for biopsy. Judgment must be exercised when deciding if an abnormality represents a separate mass or is part of the breast tissue. If in doubt, surgical excision should be performed.

During the examination the patient must be relaxed and the room adequately lighted in order to observe the breasts thoroughly. The patient should be studied while in both lying and sitting positions. In the sitting position with the arms raised above the head and clasped behind the occiput, any skin adherence or dimpling from a deeper mass will be accentuated. One should check for any change in symmetry, skin color, venous pattern, nipple elevation, or change in skin surface, including temperature.

Palpation should be carried out with the patient in both the supine and upright positions. The primary mode of evaluation should be with the patient supine, however. In this position, the breast is flattened and all the quadrants are equivalent in size. The sitting position is only to be used for palpation when it is necessary to confirm findings observed with the patient supine or to enhance nipple and subcutaneous changes. Axillary examination, however, is best performed with the patient sitting. It is essential for palpation to be performed in a gentle symmetric manner or the breast may become painful and the patient will not permit an adequate examination. The fingertips are used in concentric circles, starting and finishing at one particular area. Temperature change and alteration in skin and tissue turgor should be noted. When a mass is found, it should be evaluated for the presence or absence of a definable edge and for mobility both within the skin envelope and within the breast tissue. The consistency of the mass also must be described, and the presence of tenderness, its extension from breast tissue into the surrounding fat, and skin fixation are additional critical factors. When a mass is detected, it usually can be moved sufficiently to determine whether or not associated skin dimpling or nipple retraction is present.

Examination of the axilla is best carried out with the physician's opposite hand, with the physician standing on the opposite side of the patient. Thus, to examine the left axilla, the examiner stands on the patient's right; the right hand is used to examine the axilla while the left hand supports the patient's left arm. The hand is inserted as high in the axilla as possible and then is gently brought down along the chest wall, palpating the axillary contents between the skin and the rib cage. Comparison of the two sides is essential. The presence of normally palpable lymph nodes within the axillary fat pad is a common finding; what the physician is searching for is asymmetry of contour, fixation of nodes to the chest wall, and the presence of normal tissue above the lymph nodes. Observation of the size of the nodes, whether they are matted to each other, and whether or not they are smooth or irregular in size is essential. A statement regarding their consistency and whether or not they are actually a part of the tail of the breast is valuable information. A judgment should be made as to whether or not lymph nodes palpated in the axilla are thought to represent malignant disease.

Examination of the nipple should determine whether there is induration, excoriation, or inversion. If any of these are found and are recent, biopsy may be required. Treatment with moisturizing cream may permit a benign excoriated lesion to heal. Paget's disease, which represents an intraductal carcinoma just beneath the nipple, presents with overlying excoriation of the skin of the nipple. The surgeon should always express the nipple gently to elicit any discharge. It is also important to examine for a subareolar mass by elevating the nipple and gently compressing the tissue beneath the nipple. Subareolar masses may be present with Paget's disease or associated with nipple discharge. This is particularly true when the quadrant of the breast from which the discharge can be expressed has been identified.

Clinical TNM Staging

Several staging systems have been in use over the years to allow the physician a means of comparing one breast lesion with another and selecting therapy based on preoperative examination. Many of these staging systems have now been abandoned and the TNM system is used almost universally. The definitions of the letters T, N, and M used in the categories for carcinoma of the breast are as follows: T, primary tumors; N, regional lymph nodes; and M, distant metastasis.

Definitions of T, N, and M Categories

TIS Preinvasive carcinoma (carcinoma in situ), noninfiltrating intraductal carcinoma, or Paget's disease of the nipple with no demonstrable tumor

TO No demonstrable tumor in the breast

T1* Tumor 2 cm or less in its greatest dimension

　　T1a With no fixation to underlying pectoral fascia and/or muscle

　　T1b With fixation to underlying pectoral fascia and/or muscle

T2* Tumor more than 2 cm but not more than 5 cm in its greatest dimension

---

*Dimpling of the skin, nipple retraction, or any other skin changes except those in T4b may occur in T1, T2, or T3 without affecting the classification.

T2a With no fixation to underlying pectoral fascia and/or muscle

T2b With fixation to underlying pectoral fascia and/or muscle

T3* Tumor more than 5 cm in its greatest dimension

T3a With no fixation to underlying pectoral fascia and/or muscle

T3b With fixation to underlying pectoral fascia and/or muscle

T4 Tumor of any size with direct extension to chest wall or skin (Note: Chest wall includes ribs, intercostal muscles, and serratus anterior muscle, but not pectoral muscle)

T4a With fixation to chest wall

T4b With edema (including *peau d'orange*), ulceration of the skin of the breast, or satellite skin nodules confined to the same breast

T4c Both of above

N0 No palpable ipsilateral axillary nodes

N1 Movable ipsilateral axillary nodes

N1a Nodes not considered to contain growth

N1b Nodes considered to contain growth

N2 Ipsilateral axillary nodes considered to contain growth and fixed to one another or to other structures

N3 Ipsilateral supraclavicular or intraclavicular nodes considered to contain growth or edema of the arm

M0 No evidence of distant metastasis

M1 Distant metastasis present, including skin involvement beyond the breast area

Clinical Stage-Grouping

INVASIVE CARCINOMA

Stage I   T1a N0 or N1a
               T1b N0 or N1a   } M0

*Dimpling of the skin, nipple retraction, or any other skin changes except those in T4b may occur in T1, T2, or T3 without affecting the classification.

Stage II	T0 N1b	
	T1a N1b	
	T1b N1b	} M0
	T2a or T2b N0, N1a, or N1b	
Stage III	Any T3 with any N	
	Any T4 with any N	
	Any T with N2	} M0
	Any T with N3	
Stage IV	Any T or any N with M1	

Correlates of Physical Examination with Pathology

Mobility and sharp margination of a mass within the breast indicate benign disease. When the lesion is mobile but surrounding breast tissue moves with it, the area then becomes suspect for malignancy. As margination decreases, extension and fixation into the tissue surrounding the mass become more apparent. This is frequently confirmed with mammography. The size of malignant lesions within the breast correlates well with prognosis, smaller lesions having a better prognosis. Metastases are much more frequent with lesions greater than 5 cm.

The breast is surrounded by an envelope of fat and covered by skin. In order for the skin to be invaded, the malignancy must extend out of the breast, through the subcutaneous fat, and into the overlying skin. Skin dimpling can occur by fixation of Cooper's ligaments by the tumor or its extension. Skin dimpling as an isolated finding does not have a prognostic value, although it does tend to prove a malignant diagnosis on a clinical basis. Skin edema, however, is an important prognostic finding and always indicates severe disease. The skin lymphatics drain toward the areola and down beneath the nipple to the base of the breast. They subsequently extend through the pectoral fascia to the axilla, to the supraclavicular space, or to the internal mammary nodes. A tumor posteriorly placed within the breast can produce massive edema of the skin by blocking these lymphatic pathways. The *peau d'orange* condition occurs because the skin pores are held down by small fibrous strands that allow edema of the skin to develop between them; the breast skin then swells between the pores, thus resembling an orange peel. The more *peau d'orange* and edema, the more serious the prognosis. *Peau d'orange* for greater than one third of the breast surface makes the lesion unresectable.

Venous engorgement is a common finding in breast cancers, especially those that are far advanced. Increased blood flow to malignant tumors occurs, and if there is venous obstruction at the base of the breast, the veins on the surface of the breast will be engorged and collateral channels will then be used. Venous engorgement is particularly prominent in cystosarcoma phyllodes.

Pectoral fixation is identified by having the patient tighten her pectoral muscles by clenching her fists or hands in front of her body. Elevation of her arms above the head also will permit tightening of the pectoral muscles, and the motion of the breast on the surface of the pectoralis muscle can be determined. The presence of pectoral fixation is an important finding. Fixation to the pectoral muscle, however, does not always indicate invasion but rather can be the result of associated inflammation and adherence to the muscle. This cannot be determined until operation.

Edema of the arm indicates lymphatic obstruction in the axilla and frequently supraclavicular obstruction as well. The lymphatic network of the arm is extensive, and gross involvement is required before edema occurs. Prior x-ray therapy will increase the risk for edema. Pain in the axilla or the arm is more likely to be associated with brachial plexus involvement and is a grave sign of extensive local involvement. Pain may also represent bone involvement, and radiographs of the shoulder and arm are essential in these patients if metastases are to be found. The presence of supraclavicular nodal enlargement and associated extremity muscle wasting, anhidrosis, and drooping eyelid (Horner's syndrome) is indicative of metastatic disease and points to the spread of tumor to the supraclavicular nodes and thoracic inlet. We would not consider such patients for primary surgical treatment.

Biopsy Technique

A biopsy may be carried out in four different ways: (1) needle aspiration, (2) needle biopsy, (3) open biopsy under local anesthesia, and (4) open biopsy under general anesthesia.

Needle Aspiration

A fine needle, with a small amount of saline in the syringe for irrigation back and forth into the lesion, is utilized to obtain cytologic material. This technique has not gained wide acceptance. It is used by some authors who have extensive experience with it. Malignancy can be identified by this technique, but failure to obtain a positive diagnosis must not be construed as evidence that the lesion is categorically benign. Also, this approach cannot differentiate in-situ cancers from those that are invasive.

Needle Biopsy

Needle biopsy is usually done either with a Vim-Silverman or Tru-cut needle or, more recently, with a mechanical drill. While also not as accurate as open biopsy, it can adequately serve to establish the diagnosis. Once again, failure to obtain a positive diagnosis in a suspicious lesion does not negate the need for open biopsy. One important indication for the use of this technique is the presence of advanced disease when a large diagnostic incision in the breast is contraindicated. The more extensive the tumor, the more accurate the biopsy and the greater the likelihood of obtaining a good core of tissue. It is possible to obtain estrogen receptor protein data on needle biopsies if three or four cores are obtained. Cooperation between the surgeon and the pathologist is essential in order to obtain accurate needle biopsies.

Open Biopsy Under Local Anesthesia

The advantages of open biopsy under local anesthesia are its simplicity and the psychological advantages for the patient. By having the patient awake for the procedure, it is not necessary to prepare each patient for a possible mastectomy. Because less workup is required, the cost is greatly reduced. In addition, being able to perform these biopsies on an outpatient basis saves a great deal of time and money. Frozen section diagnosis can be obtained, and immediate plans can be arrived at, should the lesion be identified as malignant.

The disadvantage of a biopsy under local anesthesia is the pain associated with it, since most of the anesthetic is used to infiltrate the skin. It may be more difficult to biopsy more than one location, and the biopsy must, of necessity, be less extensive. When nonpalpable disease is being biopsied, general anesthesia is necessary unless the radiologist has been able to easily mark the superficial area.

Open Biopsy Under General Anesthesia

Open biopsy under general anesthesia is obviously more comfortable for the patient and allows the best definition obtainable. As just mentioned, it is usually necessary in cases of nonpalpable disease. With this type of biopsy it is possible to do a total excision of the mass, if that is desired—for example, if the planned treatment of the breast mass is to be lump removal or partial mastectomy—with subsequent radiation. If the pathologist and the surgeon, working in concert, cannot be certain of the tissue diagnosis of malignancy, then under no circumstances should mastectomy be performed at that time.

The disadvantage of open biopsy under general anesthesia is the need to prepare each patient for possible mastectomy prior to the surgery. It is less desirable to perform a second operation under general anesthesia, and if the patient will not permit a mastectomy, then every attempt should be made to perform the biopsy under local anesthesia. Since approximately only 20 percent of biopsies are positive for malignancy, the necessity of extended hospitalization and magnification of psychological problems for the patient may be enhanced if open biopsy under general anesthesia is the procedure of choice.

Nelson A. Burstein

4. Pathology of Breast Cancer

This chapter on the pathology of breast cancer discusses morphologic features that have prognostic significance. In this selected review of the literature, the emphasis is on studies that show clinical and pathologic correlation. In addition to the diagnostic and prognostic features of specific categories of breast cancer, a discussion of the pathology and biology of breast lesions in screened or high-risk patients is included.

Diagnostic and Prognostic Features of Breast Cancers

The histologic criteria for the several categories of breast cancer are discussed in detail by McDivitt and co-workers [30]. A comparison of survival rates for patients with the various tumor histologies is summarized in Table 4–1. Survival was best in patients with comedocarcinoma (74%). In contrast, the 30-year survival was least favorable in a group of patients who had a poorly differentiated scirrhous carcinoma (29%) (patients having scirrhous cancers, as a group, had a 33% 30-year survival) and in a group of patients who had infiltrating lobular (small-cell) carcinoma (34%). Patients with intermediate survival over the 30-year period were those with colloid (55%), medullary (58%), and papillary (65%) carcinomas [1]. While it is true that patients with some lesions do have better rates of survival, these lesions represent a relatively small proportion of all carcinomas of the breast. The scirrhous or infiltrating ductal carcinomas and infiltrating lobular carcinomas probably represent close to 90 percent of the carcinomas encountered clinically. Moreover, even though a lesion such as colloid or medullary carcinoma of the breast tends to be larger and have fewer lymph node metastases for tumor size, there is little in the overall natural history to justify altering therapy based purely on the histology of the lesion. These tumors still recur locally and metastasize. There is no biologic basis for isolating these tumors, on histology alone, for special therapy.

To further assess prognosis, it is useful to look beyond the histologic type of the tumor. The histologic grading of tumors

Table 4-1. Survival of Patients with Special Histology Types of Infiltrating Breast Carcinoma Compared with Ordinary Infiltrative Duct Carcinoma [1]

Histologic Type	Infiltrating Duct Carcinoma with Productive Fibrosis (scirrhous) (%)	Infiltrating Lobular Carcinoma (%)	Medullary (infiltrating) (%)	Colloid (infiltrating) (%)	Comedo-carcinomas (infiltrating) (%)	Papillary (infiltrating) (%)
Percent	78	9	4	3	5	1
Node involvement	60	60	44	32	32	17
Actuarial survival						
5 years	59	57	69	76	84	89
10 years	47	42	68	72	77	65
20 years	38	34	62	62	74	65
30 years	33	34	58	55	74	65

is based on the degree of gland formation or tubule formation in the tumor (with the most malignant having the fewest tubules) and on nuclear atypicality, which includes nuclear pleomorphism, hyperchromatism, and mitoses. The nuclear features of pleomorphism, hyperchromatism, and mitoses have more prognostic implications, oftentimes overriding a fair degree of tubule formation. Thus, the histologic grading system overlaps considerably with systems based on nuclear grade alone. In tumors in which histologic grading has been performed and the patients followed, this system proves to be useful in predicting a prognosis for groups of patients [8]. More specifically, patients with grade I carcinomas (the least malignant categories, that is, those with tubule formation and benign-appearing nuclei) had an 81 percent 5-year survival. In contrast, patients with grade II tumors had a 54 percent 5-year survival, and those with grade III tumors, 34 percent. This difference extends 20 years postoperatively in that those with grade I tumors had a 41 percent 20-year survival; grade II, 29 percent; and grade III, 21 percent. The system is useful in comparing large populations of patients as far as prognosis is concerned and is useful in the grade III and grade I tumors for evaluating prognosis. Most patients, however, fall in the grade II category, which limits the application of the grading system. Finally, while this system is useful in a general way for assessing prognosis, at present it is not appropriate or practical to deny or add therapy directed at local control or systemic cure based solely on the histologic grade of the tumor.

Tumor size is also of prognostic importance in carcinoma of the breast. In general, the larger the primary tumor, the worse the prospect for survival and the greater the probability for axillary lymph node metastasis. A recent large series of patients with operative breast cancers [13] was evaluated concerning size of the tumor, which was then correlated with nodal metastasis and 5-year survival. The distribution of the patients' tumors was what might be expected in the general population; namely, 5 percent of the tumors were under 1 cm in diameter, and 28 percent exceeded 4 cm in diameter, with the other 67 percent falling in between. There was a relationship between tumor size and node status. In patients whose lymph nodes were negative for tumor, the average tumor size was 2.7 cm; in a group with one to three positive nodes, the average tumor was 2.9 cm; and in a group of patients with four or more positive nodes, the median tumor size was 3.3 cm.

This slight relationship between tumor size and nodal metastasis has to be accepted with reservation as far as prognosis is concerned since as many as 22 percent of the patients with tumors less than 1 cm had axillary metastasis. When the 5-year survival was evaluated as a function of size alone, patients with tumors less than 1 cm in diameter had a survival rate of 82 percent; and those with tumors of 1 to 1.9 cm, 78 percent. Those having tumors exceeding 6 cm in diameter had a survival of 57 percent. If one looks at tumor size but then corrects for node status, however, size becomes less significant. In the group with negative nodes, patients with small tumors and large tumors did approximately as well over 5 years. However, in the group of patients with more than four positive axillary nodes, mortality correlated with tumor size. This recent report [13] confirms other studies that show that tumor size alone does not necessarily correlate with survival. An insight given by this study is the importance of knowing the status of nodal metastasis in the axilla as a basis for making a decision on the form of local or systemic therapy; thus, measuring the size of the tumor does not obviate the need for an axillary sampling procedure.

Tumor size is important when discussing the concept of minimal breast carcinoma. This term was introduced by Gallagher and Martin [20] to describe a group of carcinomas that were in situ or invasive but formed a mass that was no larger than 0.5 cm. Others have used the term to refer to the same small invasive cancers but have included carcinomas of favorable type, such as medullary or colloid, regardless of tumor size. A third group of pathologists prefers to separate the in-situ carcinomas that may be present in the small lesions from small invasive carcinomas. In this chapter the term *minimal carcinoma* will be used to refer only to those lesions that are invasive and less than 1 cm in diameter. I believe this is an important distinction, since patients with lesions of this size can still have up to 20 percent of the lymph nodes be positive. In the other small in-situ carcinomas, the biologic malignancy is more difficult to prove since they lack invasion and metastasis. This point will be discussed later in the chapter.

Invasion or noninvasion of blood vessels is another feature

of the primary tumor that may have prognostic significance. The usual method for evaluating invasion is by use of an elastic tissue stain to look for a tumor that is penetrating vessel walls and forming tumor thrombi in vessels. Some [15] report blood vessel invasion as a poor prognostic sign in all patients, independent of node status; others [18] only in patients with negative lymph nodes; still others [19] only in patients who have positive nodes; and, finally, there are reports [25] showing that there is no significance to blood vessel invasion. One of the difficulties in assessing these reports is the variation in incidence of blood vessel invasion reported among many authors. This may be due in part to the difficulty of distinguishing the blood vessel from the wall of the duct that contains extensive elastic fibers. Although it would be unwise to dismiss blood vessel invasion as a meaningless feature of tumors, its presence seems to add little additional information when assessing prognosis, particularly when this information is compared with histologic type of tumor, histologic grade, and the presence or absence of axillary node metastasis.

The inflammatory reaction within the tumor may be of significance in assessing prognosis. Certainly the medullary carcinoma has a better prognosis with less intense plasmacytic infiltrate. However, when an intense plasma cell infiltrate is seen in association with the usual scirrhous carcinoma, this feature has minimal prognostic significance. It has been found recently that the presence of perivenous lymphoid cell infiltration and a diffuse lymphoid cell infiltrative tumor appear to have prognostic significance. There appears to be an association of diffuse lymphocytic infiltrate with tumors of a more malignant nuclear grade and follicular hyperplasia of the lymph node. In addition, a perivenous lymphoid infiltrate seems to be a positive prognostic factor similar to sinus histiocytosis in the lymph node [7]. These inflammatory and possibly immunologic type reactions of the host to the primary tumor may prove to have prognostic significance and should be considered in future studies.

Inflammatory Carcinoma

Inflammatory carcinoma of the breast, because of its special requirements for therapy, deserves specific mention. It represents from 1 to 4 percent of all breast cancers, and its major feature is an erythematous discoloration of the skin, usually associated with edema and extending across at least one third of the breast. The skin has a brawny, pitted appearance and texture (called *peau d'orange*). Erythema can also have a distinct raised margin reminiscent of erysipela. Axillary node enlargement is almost invariable. The term inflammatory carcinoma itself is a clinical diagnosis and not a pathologic one. The appearance is due in the majority of cases to tumor extension into and obstruction of the dermal lymphatics. In some cases with the same clinical appearance, tumor cells in dermal lymphatics cannot be demonstrated. There is some controversy in the literature as to whether invasion of dermal lymphatics by tumor is necessary for the diagnosis of inflammatory carcinoma. A recent series of inflammatory carcinoma patients, with tumor involving extensive areas of the breast, had the same poor prognosis, independent of documentation of tumor cells within the dermal lymphatics [32].

The significance of the dermal lymphatic invasion in the context of inflammatory carcinoma represents a local disseminated process. However, isolated dermal involvement by tumor in the absence of the clinical constellation described just previously should not be included when considering inflammatory carcinoma as a diagnosis, particularly in the absence of involved axillary nodes. On the other hand, not all inflammatory carcinomas will have easily demonstrable dermal lymphatic invasion nor, for that matter, need all tumors with lymphatic invasion be called inflammatory carcinoma in the absence of the usual clinical constellation of findings; many T3 lesions will show lymphatic involvement without any clinical inflammatory signs. Finally, tumors with inflammation—mainly lymphocytes, plasma cells, and other inflammatory reactive cells within a carcinoma— while representing some form of host response to the tumor, should not be placed in the category of inflammatory carcinoma.

Paget's Disease

Paget's disease of the breast was first described as an edematous eruption involving the nipple and areola that subsequently develops a scirrhous cancer. The cells in Paget's disease are large and ovoid, with an abundant clear- to pale-staining opaque cytoplasm. There is a large, round, ovoid nucleus. The most frequent location is in the malpighian layer of the epidermis. As the skin matures, the Paget cells move toward the surface. The biologic significance of these changes is an invariable association with a deeper in-situ or infiltrating carcinoma of the mammary duct. The presence of a mass lesion associated with Paget's disease carries an unfavorable prognosis. In contrast, even when there is invasive carcinoma, a nonpalpable lesion in association with Paget's disease is believed to indicate a favorable prognosis. In one series of 43 patients with Paget's disease, a clinical mass was present in 24; of these, only 6 survived 5 years. Of 19 patients without a clinical mass, 13 survived 5 years [30].

Carcinoma of the Male Breast

Carcinoma of the male breast is unusual. All histologic types have been reported, with the possible exception of lobular carcinoma, although a small-cell infiltrating variety has been seen. As in the female, about 85 percent of male breast cancers are of the infiltrating ductal variety, but medullary, papillary, and mucinous colloid carcinomas have also been reported. Some clinical presentations such as inflammatory carcinoma and Paget's disease are also seen. The survival rate is comparable to that of females when corrected for the stage of presentation. Histologic grading carries with it the same significance as it does in female breast cancer. If taken as a group, however, male breast cancer patients tend to have poorer survival than women, probably because of the advanced stage at which the disease presents [9].

The relationship between gynecomastia and male breast cancer is unclear [40]. Gynecomastia can be demonstrated in males with breast cancer, and ductal epithelium may be proliferative and even demonstrate atypia or carcinoma in situ. It is true that patients with Klinefelter's syndrome have an increased incidence of carcinoma of the breast and they also have gynecomastia. In other studies, gynecomastia can be associated with lesions in breast cancer patients. Despite all this, however, it is difficult to prove that the carcinoma arises out of the gynecomastia and that the gynecomastia is unique or, for that matter, is a significant marker for the subsequent development of carcinoma.

Cystosarcoma Phyllodes

Another malignant neoplasm within the breast is cystosarcoma phyllodes. These large lesions have a characteristic leaflike, cystic gross appearance and contain epithelium and fibrous stromal components, with a greater degree of stromal cellularity than the usual fibroadenoma. This increase in stromal cellularity is often the distinguishing feature between the fibroadenoma and the cystosarcoma phyllodes.

Several studies have attempted to look at histologic features that would predict the potential for malignancy of these lesions. One such study by Norris and Taylor [31] reviewed 94 patients with this diagnosis. The tumor recurred in 28 patients and caused death in 15 patients with metastatic disease. Most of the recurrences were within 2 years of the initial treatment, and those who died did so within 6 years. No tumors less than 4 cm in diameter or having less than three mitotic figures per 10 high power fields proved fatal. Other features that were important for a low risk of recurrence or death were an expanding, somewhat encapsulated, pushing margin (only 1 death in 39 patients) or minimal atypicality of the stromal cells (2 deaths in 30 patients). Unfortunately, as is apparent from these statistics, no one feature was totally reliable, and a clear separation between benign and malignant tumors could not be made. There were lesions with minimal mitoses and minimal cellular atypicality that had rapid clinical courses. Lymph nodes were enlarged in 17 percent of the patients, and metastases occurred in only 3 of the 94 patients. When metastasis occurred, it tended to be to the lungs.

In another study [33], 42 patients with this diagnosis were evaluated again to see what predictive features might be developed. In this study, tumor size was not a significant variable; however, an "infiltrative" versus a "pushing" border still proved to be a useful predictive feature. Again, stromal atypicality and mitotic activity were relatively reliable indicators of clinical behavior. The authors reemphasize that the tumor can recur locally, independent of these prognostic features, and that these tumors tend to metastasize systemically, often to the lungs, rather than to the axilla.

Multicentric Invasive Carcinomas
In recent years, due to the reintroduction of partial mastectomies and more conservative primary management procedures, along with the recognized value of assessing the risk of malignancy in the opposite breast, it has become important to study

the distribution of minimal and occult carcinomas. In a study analyzing 904 breasts removed for infiltrating carcinoma [16], carcinoma was found in quadrants away from the primary tumor mass in 121 patients, or over 13 percent of patients. Of these, 37 were infiltrative carcinomas while 84 were in situ. Of the multicentric invasive carcinomas, many were found in more than one quadrant. Factors that seem to be associated with multicentricity were a prominent intraductal component of the primary tumor, carcinoma in situ in the vicinity of the tumor, nipple involvement by carcinoma, and a tumor size greater than 5 cm. Multicentric invasive carcinoma was particularly common with the infiltrating lobular type. Another study [35] attempted to assess the efficiency of partial mastectomy in removing microscopic residual carcinoma. In mastectomy specimens having invasive carcinoma, the primary tumor with a 2 cm margin was excised and the new "resection margin" and remaining breast were then evaluated. If the tumor was less than 1 cm in diameter, residual infiltrating carcinoma was present in the remaining breast 11 percent of the time, and in-situ carcinoma an additional 22 percent. When the primary tumor exceeded 4 cm in diameter, 43 percent of the breasts had residual infiltrating carcinoma and 11 percent had in-situ carcinoma.

Bilateral Disease
In addition to multifocal ipsilateral carcinoma of the breast, certain morphologic findings may be associated with bilateral disease. It is known from a follow-up study in 1458 women with ipsilateral carcinoma of the breast that 94 new primaries were found in the opposite breast over a period of 20 years [34]. In this study the annual incidence of carcinoma was constant at approximately 7 cases per year per 1000 patients at risk; this number was about five times greater than that of the general population. In addition, it appeared that bilaterality depended on menopausal status, since premenopausal patients (those under the age of 50) had a greater risk of developing bilateral carcinoma than those who developed their first carcinoma after that age. The pathologic parameters of importance for bilaterality include histologic type and multifocality. The usual scirrhous, infiltrating ductal carcinoma has little association with bilaterality. In contrast, medullary carcinoma, colloid carcinoma, lobular carcinoma, and intraductal carcinomas pose

a significantly increased risk. Multifocal carcinoma in the first breast also carries with it a greater risk for bilaterality.

Of particular interest in the question of bilaterality is the particular significance of the diagnosis of infiltrating lobular (small-cell) carcinoma. As we will discuss subsequently, there is an increased risk to the patient with the diagnosis of lobular carcinoma in situ, both in the breast from which the biopsy was obtained and on the contralateral side. Some authors, for example, Fechner [12], feel that the infiltrating small-cell carcinoma unassociated with in-situ changes also increases the risk of contralateral disease. Others [14] point out that this diagnosis in the absence of in-situ or intraductal changes carries with it no greater risk for the contralateral primary than infiltrating scirrhous carcinoma. If one includes, however, lobular carcinoma arising in association with lobular carcinoma in situ and intraductal proliferation, then the bilaterality rate either with simultaneous discovery or subsequent development of a lesion can approach 50 percent.

As a result of these findings, various authors recommend additional surgical procedures ranging from mirror image biopsy or outer quadrant biopsy to contralateral mastectomy. When these procedures are performed, a significant number of in-situ and an occasional invasive carcinoma may be discovered.

In an attempt to assess the risk of a synchronous second primary in the opposite breast and to find early in-situ changes or carcinoma, Urban and co-workers [42] performed outer quadrant biopsies as well as mirror-image biopsies in the breast opposite the one in which a carcinoma had been discovered. Of 339 biopsies, 14 percent contained carcinoma, one third of which were infiltrating and two thirds noninfiltrating. The positive biopsies were more frequent (20%) in patients with in-situ carcinoma as compared to those with purely invasive carcinomas without in-situ changes (8%). Some authors feel that the risk of bilaterality is sufficient in all cases of breast cancer to suggest a prophylactic mastectomy, if there is a good chance for survival. In one such study [26], 71 specimens contained 11 carcinomas and 5 were invasive. Whether or not the risks of bilaterality are great enough to justify this radical approach to therapy is unclear. Other considerations may be important; for example, if a family history is positive, the incidence of bilateral disease is much greater.

It is true that the carcinomas found by empirical biopsies are usually at an earlier stage, being both smaller and often in situ. However, one has to question the biologic significance of these lesions. In the Urban [42] series, only 1 of 17 had metastasized to the axillary lymph nodes. It is possible, although unproved, that all of these in-situ lesions would go on to become invasive carcinoma.

In summary, the most useful prognostic features in primary breast cancer are the histologic type and histologic grade of the carcinoma. Tumor size has some predictive value. The incidence of multifocality is related to tumor size, histologic type, and the presence of adjacent intraductal carcinoma. Bilaterality is related to histologic type (i.e., seen less frequently in the infiltrating ductal cancer), the presence of intraductal or lobular carcinoma in situ, and the menopausal status of the patient (premenopausal being more significant). The clinical and biologic significance of bilateral, occult carcinomas found in blind sampling of the opposite breast is unclear.

Patterns of Spread

The presence and extent of metastasis to axillary lymph node is one of the most important variables for predicting the survival of patients with breast cancer. The extent of axillary lymph node involvement has classically been defined by dividing the axillary dissection into thirds, using the pectoralis minor muscle as a reference point. The current practice in surgery does not always provide the pathologist with an axillary sample with its usual landmark. However, it is still practical to count the number of positive nodes with some general reference as to their distance and position in relation to the anatomic lymphatic spread in the breast. If no axillary lymph nodes are involved with carcinoma, the 20-year survival is approximately 65 percent. If those nodes in the lower third (closest to the breast) are involved (level one), the survival rate drops to 38 percent; for those at level two (intermediate distance), 30 percent; and if the highest (most distal) level (level three) is involved, the survival rate drops to 12 percent [30]. Survival decreases as the number of positive nodes increases, with a large downward change occurring when four or more nodes become positive [39].

When one discusses the positivity or negativity of nodes, one must comment on the significance of occult or microscopic foci in these nodes. It has been shown that if one were to serially section lymph nodes that were originally called negative by the pathologist, one would find additional tumor deposits in approximately one third of these nodes. Patients who were "node negative" would become "node positive." It is interesting, however, that as a population, *these* previously node-negative patients do not have the poor survival rate usually associated with grossly positive axillary nodes [38]. Perhaps the bulk of the metastasis is more important.

In a study of the axillary metastases of 227 patients, a division into node-positive patients and into those who had metastases less than 2 mm was made. It is interesting that those patients with micrometastases, in contrast to those with macrometastases, showed surprisingly good survival. In fact, if level one was involved, the 8-year postmastectomy survival rate was approximately that of those who had no axillary metastases. On the other hand, patients who had level one macrometastasis had a less favorable survival than those who only had micrometastasis at level three [24]. When 105 of these same patients were followed for 14 years, the group with micrometastases maintained their improved prognosis with survivals of 85 percent at 10 years and 77 percent at 14 years [4].

Thus, it appears that the bulk of the metastasis as well as the number of nodes involved may be biologically important, at least in the short follow-up. It is certainly possible that at 20 or 30 years these small metastases may take on greater significance and that the survival statistics at that time may not appear as favorable. However, if one were looking at short-term responses to either surgery or some form of adjuvant therapy, it certainly would be important to distinguish between positive lymph nodes with micrometastasis and those with macrometastatic lesions.

Another consideration that becomes important in evaluating the axilla is the extranodal extension of tumor. Apparently, if tumor extends outside the capsule of the lymph node, there is an increased rate of treatment failure. This effect appears most prominent in those patients with less than three involved axillary nodes. It has little significance in patients with four or more involved nodes. This unfavorable effect was on survival and did not influence the interval between surgery and recurrence or the distribution of the recurrence or metastasis [28].

There have been many attempts to evaluate variations in the axillary lymph nodes of patients with carcinoma of the breast that may correlate with prognosis. One of the earliest parameters to be evaluated was that of sinus histiocytosis. Some feel that the presence of sinus histiocytosis correlates with improved prognosis [10]; others claim that it has no effect. From a practical standpoint, this evaluation does not appear to have reached the level at which one can stratify patients for some clinical study or therapy plan based on the presence, absence, or degree of sinus histiocytosis. In other studies, the lymphocyte reactive patterns within the nodes have been classified as either lymphocyte predominant, germinal center predominant, or lymphocyte depleted or unstimulated. The lymphocyte predominant pattern is thought to be the most favorable, with the least favorable being lymphocyte depleted [41]. Others applying the same classification, however, see no evidence that this provides a prognostic indicator and observe similar short-term failure in all groups of patients [17].

In summary, the most significant feature of lymph node pathology is the presence or absence of metastatic carcinoma. As discussed above, the other histologic patterns that are seen in association with carcinoma may represent some underlying immunologic tumor-host interaction, although they are presently of little practical clinical significance. The presence of lymph node metastasis in a carcinoma of the breast probably should not be construed as a measure of the "lateness" or "earliness" of the tumor, particularly when early and late may be applied to patient or physician delay or time in which the tumor has remained subclinical. Rather, it might be better considered as an independent variable that carries with it a considerable association with prognosis because it represents a feature that may combine both the tumor-host relationship from an immunologic standpoint (the tumor is residing in a lymph node and is not destroyed by it) and the tumor's ability to invade lymphatics or blood vessels and survive and multiply in this foreign environment.

Occasionally, a metastatic carcinoma is present in an axillary lymph node in the absence of a clinically apparent primary in the breast. Obviously, a breast primary must be pursued with mammography, physical examination, and other indirect approaches. When this situation has been studied, over two-thirds of patients who subsequently had mastectomies were found to have had occult carcinomas of the breast, most measuring less than 2 cm in diameter [3]. It is important to remember, however, that carcinomas can arise in the axillary tail of the breast, which can cause confusion since the initial axillary biopsy may remove the primary. This could pose a problem, particularly with a tumor with an intense lymphocytic infiltration. Other primary sites have been known to produce metastases to the axilla as their presenting finding; these include lung, stomach, and pancreas.

It is important to remember that while the estrogen receptor assay has currently attained some status in predicting hormone responsiveness in breast tumors, it has limited value in evaluating the axillary node. If tumor in the node contains estrogen receptor (see Chap. 5), then the breast certainly rates high consideration, since significant levels of receptor are rarely seen in other tumors. However, even if the metastatic carcinoma does not contain estrogen-binding protein, the breast is still the most likely possibility as a site of the primary tumor. It is of interest that in the small series of patients with occult breast carcinoma presenting with an axillary mass, survival seemed to be better than in patients presenting with a clinically apparent carcinoma of the breast with axillary node involvement. Survival did not seem to be affected by whether or not the primary tumor was found.

Distribution and metastasis of breast cancer does not correspond to the cardiac output distribution. In fact, it is quite apparent that the differing incidence of metastases in bone, lungs, pleura, liver, and brain indicates the importance of certain local site factors in determining where metastasis develops. The sites of metastasis at autopsy in patients with breast cancer are illustrated in Table 4–2. Of particular interest is a relatively high amount of metastasis to the adrenal glands and the ovary. In some series examining surgical adrenalectomy and oophorectomy in the treatment of metastatic breast cancer, 39 percent of the adrenals and 29 percent of the ovaries were involved with breast carcinoma [27]. This is not surprising in light of the known hormone dependence of many breast carcinomas.

Table 4-2. Frequency of Breast Cancer Metastases at Necropsy (100 Cases) [27]

50–75%	25–40%	10–15%
Lungs	Adrenals	Pancreas
Pleura	Ovaries	Kidney
Bones	Skin	Spleen
Liver	Diaphragm	Uterus
Lymph nodes	Pericardium	Intestine
		Heart
		Thyroid
		Brain

Source: G. Lumb and D. H. Mackenzie. The incidence of metastases in adrenal glands and ovaries removed for carcinoma of the breast. *Cancer* 12:521, 1959.

While there is a suggestion in some series that patients with ovarian or adrenal metastasis have a greater propensity for response to the ablative endocrine procedures, the predictive value of ovarian or adrenal metastasis is minimal. In patients with ovarian or adrenal metastasis, there is little evidence of autocastration or autoadrenalectomy, although in patients with adrenal metastases there may be a decreased adrenal reserve, and in pituitary metastases diabetes insipidus can occur. Metastases to the lung are fairly common and usually pose no diagnostic problems; however, these metastases may not occur until after a period of many years. In these situations, we have found an estrogen receptor assay on solitary or multiple tissue samples from the lung very helpful in raising the possibility of recurrent carcinoma of the breast. Gastric metastases, while uncommon, do occur, and here again an estrogen receptor assay may be helpful in suggesting the breast as the primary tumor.

Problems with High-Risk and Screened Populations

Mammography has helped to extend our knowledge of breast carcinoma in two ways. First, it has provided pathologic specimens evaluated as positive or suspicious by mammographic study but clinically not palpable. In addition, it has extended to the pathologist the opportunity of finding small lesions in specimens submitted for gross evaluation and microscopic sampling. This section will not discuss the pathology of palpable lesions that were mammographically suspicious, but rather those lesions that were biopsied solely on the basis of a positive mammogram. In the study of 80 breast biopsies taken for these reasons, Rosen and associates [37] found that 12 (15%) of these biopsy specimens contained carcinoma. Of the 12 carcinomas, 10 were intraductal (1 contained an area of microinvasion), and 2 showed lobular carcinoma in situ. Invasive carcinoma appeared in fewer than 2 percent of the 80 breast biopsies; intraductal papillomatosis was present in 23 percent, and other benign lesions were seen in 43 percent of the biopsy specimens. The biologic significance of these intraductal and lobular carcinomas in situ will be discussed. In a similar series of 54 patients with nonpalpable but mammographically suspicious lesions, 14 (25%) had occult carcinomas [5]. It is unclear from this report, however, whether they were invasive or in situ.

Aspiration biopsy with cytology plays a useful role in the diagnosis of breast cancer. The usefulness of this technique was demonstrated in a recent study [44] in which aspiration cytology was performed on 2772 breast masses, all of which underwent subsequent biopsies. Of 1745 histologically malignant tumors, 1539 (88%) had a cytologic diagnosis of malignancy, 54 (3%) were diagnosed probably malignant, and 63 (4%) were false negative. An additional 89 (5%) had inadequate smears for diagnosis. Of the 1027 benign lesions, 89% had a benign cytologic diagnosis. Only 3 (0.3%) were false positive. Cancer was suggested in 42 patients (4%), and the smears were inadequate for cytology in 66 cases (6.4%). Sampling error apparently played a role in the very small or large carcinomas in generating the false negative cytologies. Also, when tumors were well differentiated, difficulty arose in the diagnosis of malignancy by cytologic means. It is apparent from this report that cytology in experienced hands is reliable for the diagnosis of carcinoma when aspirations are positive but should be ignored if they are inadequate or if no malignant cells are seen.

A similar report by Hajdu and Melamed [22] points out the strength and limitations of cytologic diagnostic techniques. In it, the importance of establishing standards for the cytologic diagnosis of malignancy is stressed so that one eliminates false positives and accepts many false negative reports. In Hajdu and Melamed's series of 315 breast aspirations, all of their diagnoses of malignancy were confirmed at biopsy. However, of 141 aspirations that were diagnosed as negative or inadequate, carcinoma was subsequently seen in 45 percent of the patients. Again, this technique is useful when it is positive but should not be relied on when it is negative. There are many examples of patients with small palpable carcinomas in which therapy was delayed as a result of a negative or benign diagnosis on aspiration cytology. Finally, aspiration cytology, either for the diagnosis of carcinoma or for indication of need for subsequent biopsy in the case of the negative cytologies, can only be used with confidence at institutions in which there is a large volume of breast carcinoma and a pathology department interested and experienced in the use of aspiration cytology for the diagnosis of carcinoma.

Differentiating Preinvasive Carcinoma from Benign Disease

In recent years, through the introduction of diagnostic techniques such as mammography and the greater awareness on the part of the public and physicians of the importance of early diagnosis and of the curability of carcinoma of the breast, the pathologist has been presented with the opportunity to diagnose breast cancer earlier in its clinical course. As a result, he has been faced with the problems of differentiating preinvasive carcinomas from proliferative forms of benign breast disease, which can appear quite similar. The problems for the pathologist might best be divided into two general categories. The first involves an in-situ carcinoma, the carcinoma before it invades: how does it differ from a small invasive carcinoma from a biologic standpoint? Second, in what setting of benign breast disease does carcinoma of the breast arise?

Carcinoma In Situ. In beginning the discussion of carcinoma in situ, I think it is important to point out that all carcinomas must arise from an atypical and malignant transformation within the breast. Moreover, if one could diagnose and treat these early carcinomatous changes in the breast at their preinvasive stage, one should be able to prevent the development of carcinoma and affect the mortality due to breast cancer. That is the philosophical basis of screening.

Morphologically, however, in-situ carcinoma is a contradiction in terms. Carcinoma is a malignant neoplasm that invades and has the ability to metastasize and often kill the host. In-situ carcinoma, in contrast, does not invade and does not metastasize or result in death of the host. These in-situ lesions in ducts and lobules were originally described in association with a carcinoma. Many times the same cells, or very similar cells, that were present in the invading tumor were seen within the adjacent ducts and lobules. Since they looked the same, had not invaded, and were seen in association with the invasive carcinoma, it seemed reasonable to label these lesions as in-situ carcinoma.

Further studies supported this concept, including studies in which the in-situ lesions were only locally treated and the patients subsequently developed invasive carcinoma in the adjacent and surrounding breast tissue. These studies and those that will be discussed subsequently point to a circularity in the logic of defining in-situ carcinoma. The lesions removed from the breast and labeled in-situ carcinoma are embedded in paraffin and safely stored in a subbasement of some pathology department, while it is the adjacent breast that gives rise to the invasive carcinoma. The association of in-situ carcinoma with invasive carcinoma—the association that generates the name *in-situ*—also generates one of the major problems in assessing its biology. If a tumor arises either in a short period (months) or over a slightly longer period, an author may say that the invasive carcinoma that developed in association with in-situ carcinoma was already there in a similar state that was not clinically apparent or that the surgeon may have missed the main lesion in his biopsy.

It is clear from a review of these articles that in-situ carcinomas have an increased likelihood of being associated with breast cancer. There seem to be varying degrees of increased risk of subsequently developing carcinoma in the tissues adjacent to the biopsy and elsewhere in the same breast. Moreover, breast cancer patients probably have a greater risk of developing a primary invasive carcinoma in the opposite breast than do women in the general population. Finally, these in-situ carcinoma changes, both ductal and lobular, tend to be multifocal within the breast.

As with any disease process that is sampled in a variety of ways under a variety of circumstances and followed in patients in different manners, the degree of risk to the same breast and opposite breast varies in many series [29, 30]. Retrospective studies that review previously diagnosed benign breast biopsies show that in those patients with in-situ carcinomas that were removed, there is minimal, if any, risk for subsequent development of carcinoma of the breast [2, 21, 43]. Other studies, both prospective and retrospective, show an increased risk that may be more than five times that of the general population [23, 36]. In approaching the patient with in-situ carcinoma, one is faced with a biologic dilemma; that is, one can treat aggressively an in-situ lesion that has definite but limited biologic malignant potential in any individual patient, or one can undertreat and follow the patient to let the breast tissue neighboring the in-situ lesion develop a less curable invasive carcinoma.

Cystic Disease. If the relationship between in-situ carcinoma and malignant invasive carcinoma of the breast is unclear, then the relationship between benign breast disease and invasive carcinoma is even less certain [29, 30]. The term *cystic disease* of the breast is as much a frustration to pathologists in their attempt to categorize benign breast disease as it is to surgeons and other interested parties attempting to glean predictive information from pathology reports. Unfortunately, most breast biopsy material that is not clearly from a fibroadenoma or an in-situ or invasive carcinoma appears to be placed in this diagnostic category of cystic disease. Frustration is the only thing that can be generated if one tries to predict or associate a subsequent malignant event with the presence or absence of this "disease."

Cystic disease probably represents a mixture of normal and abnormal physiologic changes within the breast; fibrous reactions and reparative phenomena associated with injury, senescence, or regeneration; and a more proliferative form of a process that may be associated with malignant sequela. If one were to look at breast specimens taken at autopsy, close to 50 percent would show changes that easily should be diagnosed as cystic disease.

When one attempts to look for types or categories of cystic disease associated with the subsequent or concomitant development of malignancy, most studies emphasize the proliferative forms. One particularly mentioned is intraductal papillomatosis with extensive hyperplasia in many of the large ducts and other forms of intraductal hyperplasia. Also, lobular proliferations with filling of the lobules and terminal branches of the ducts with proliferating atypical cells have been associated with malignancy. The morphology of these lesions is well described

[30]. However, the biology of these lesions is unclear. It is true that, in retrospective studies of patients who subsequently develop carcinoma of the breast, there is a significant association of these proliferative and atypically proliferative lesions with subsequent invasive carcinoma [6, 11].

All of the problems in interpretation that we alluded to in our discussion of in-situ carcinoma and invasive carcinoma hold true when dealing with the proliferative forms of cystic disease as well. It is made even more complicated by the fact that there is a looser association between invasive carcinoma and cystic disease. Here again, the physician is faced with a similar biologic indeterminacy of the pathologic lesion and a clinical dilemma. He can treat aggressively and probably overtreat the majority of patients with this particular pathology, or he can undertreat—hopefully following these patients as closely as a high-risk patient—at the risk of having the patients develop invasive carcinomas that will be less amenable to therapy. Unfortunately, at present there are few, if any, nonmorphologic ways to approach the problem. As is the case with in-situ carcinoma, the invasive carcinoma may be adjacent to the proliferative cystic disease that is biopsied and be missed at the initial biopsy. As is also the case with in-situ carcinomas with proliferative cystic disease, there tends to be a multifocal quality to the disease process; moreover, the opposite breast is similarly at risk. Although proliferative cystic disease is sufficient to place the patient in a high-risk category, it, by itself, does not require therapy for invasive carcinoma.

Research Goals

In this technologically limitless medical environment, it is tempting to refine our screening techniques to find the smallest possible carcinoma and permit intervention in the course of a patient's disease at the earliest possible stage. While these research goals are on the surface quite laudatory, they raise certain problems that are difficult to deal with from a morphologic and biologic standpoint. One can conceive of the "early" carcinoma as being like the "late" carcinoma, only smaller. As a matter of fact, many of these early invasive carcinomas are biologically quite late in that they have already metastasized to nodes. The early carcinomas we would like to find are the premalignant lesions and in-situ carcinomas. It should be appreciated, however, that the early diagnosis of these atypical and premalignant lesions, most of which will not later develop into biologically significant malignancies, may have little impact on the overall effect of therapy directed at breast cancer in general.

In summary, the major morphologic problems that arise in screened populations relate to the biologic indeterminacy of the lesions called carcinoma in situ and proliferative cystic disease. The risk of concurrent and subsequent invasive carcinoma is increased with both processes, the opposite breast having the same risk as the side from which the biopsy was taken. However, in the majority of cases, the biopsy procedure itself is curative. Even the presence of epithelial atypicality or in-situ carcinoma in the remaining breast tissue away from the biopsy site may have limited biologic significance.

References

1. Adair, F., Berg, J., Jouber, L., et al. Long-term follow-up of the breast cancer patient: The 30 year report. *Cancer* 33:1145, 1974.
2. Ashikari, R., Huvos, A. G., and Snyder, R. E. Prospective study of non-infiltrating carcinoma of the breast. *Cancer* 39:435, 1977.
3. Ashikari, R., Rosen, P. P., Urban, J. A., et al. Breast cancer presenting as an axillary mass. *Ann. Surg.* 183:415, 1976.
4. Attiyeh, F. F., Jensen, M., Huvos, A. G., et al. Axillary micrometastasis and macrometastasis in carcinoma of the breast. *Surg. Gynecol. Obstet.* 144:839, 1977.
5. Bauermeister, D. E., and McClure, H. H. Specimen radiography—a mandatory adjunct to mammography. *Am. J. Clin. Pathol.* 59:782, 1973.
6. Black, M. M., Barclay, T. H. C., Cutler, S. J., et al. Association of atypical characteristics of benign breast lesions with subsequent risk of breast cancer. *Cancer* 29:338, 1972.
7. Black, M. M., Barclay, T. H. C., and Hankey, B. F. Prognosis in breast cancer utilizing histologic characteristics of the primary tumor. *Cancer* 36:2048, 1975.
8. Bloom, H. J. G., and Richardson, W. W. Histological grading and prognosis in breast cancer. A study of 1409 cases of which 359 have been followed for 15 years. *Br. J. Cancer* 11:359, 1957.
9. Crichlow, R. W. Breast cancer in males. *Breast* 2:12, 1976.
10. Cutler, S. J., Black, M. M., Mork, T., et al. Further observations on prognostic factors in cancer of the female breast. *Cancer* 24:653, 1969.
11. Davis, H. H., Simons, M., and Davis, J. B. Cystic disease of the breast: Relationship to carcinoma. *Cancer* 17:957, 1964.
12. Fechner, R. E. Infiltrating lobular carcinoma without lobular carcinoma in situ. *Cancer* 29:1539, 1972.

13. Fisher, B., Slack, N. H., Bross, I. D. J., et al. Cancer of the breast: Size of neoplasm and prognosis. *Cancer* 24:1071, 1969.
14. Fisher, E. R., and Fisher, B. Lobular carcinoma of the breast: An overview. *Ann. Surg.* 185:377, 1977.
15. Fisher, E. R., Gregorio, R. M., and Fisher, B. The pathology of invasive breast cancer. *Cancer* 36:1, 1975.
16. Fisher, E. R., Gregorio, R. M., Redmond, C., et al. Pathologic findings from the national surgical adjuvant breast project (Protocol No. 4): I. Observations concerning the multicentricity of mammary cancer. *Cancer* 35:247, 1975.
17. Fisher, E. R., Gregorio, R. M., Redmond, C., et al. Pathologic findings from the national surgical adjuvant breast project (Protocol No. 4): II. The significance of regional node histology other than sinus histiocytosis in invasive mammary cancer. *Am. J. Clin. Pathol.* 65:21, 1976.
18. Friedell, G. H., Betts, A., and Sommers, S. C. The prognostic value of blood vessel invasion and lymphocytic infiltrates in breast carcinoma. *Cancer* 18:164, 1965.
19. Friedell, G. H., Goldenberg, I. S., Masnyk, I. J., et al. Identification of breast cancer patients with high risk of early recurrence after radical mastectomy: I. Description of study. *J. Natl. Cancer Inst.* 53:603, 1974.
20. Gallager, H. S., and Martin, J. E. An orientation to the concept of minimal breast cancer. *Cancer* 28:1505, 1971.
21. Haagensen, C. D., Lane, N., Lattes, R., et al. Lobular neoplasia (so-called lobular carcinoma in situ) of the breast. *Cancer* 42:737, 1978.
22. Hajdu, S. I., and Melamed, M. R. The diagnostic value of aspiration smears. *Am. J. Clin. Pathol.* 59:350, 1973.
23. Hutter, R. V. P., and Foote, F. W. Lobular carcinoma in situ. Long term follow-up. *Cancer* 24:1081, 1969.
24. Huvos, A. G., Hutter, R. V. P., and Berg, J. W. Significance of axillary macrometastases and micrometastases in mammary cancer. *Ann. Surg.* 173:44, 1971.
25. Kister, S. J., Sommers, S. C., Haagensen, C. D., et al. Re-evaluation of blood-vessel invasion as a prognostic factor in carcinoma of the breast. *Cancer* 19:1213, 1966.
26. Leis, H. P., Jr., Mersheimer, W. L., Black, N. N., et al. The second breast. *N.Y. J. Med.* 65:2460, 1965.
27. Lumb, G., and Mackenzie, D. H. The incidence of metastases in adrenal glands and ovaries removed for carcinoma of the breast. *Cancer* 12:521, 1959.
28. Mambo, N. C., and Gallager, H. S. Carcinoma of the breast. The prognostic significance of extranodal extension of axillary disease. *Cancer* 39:2280, 1977.
29. McDivitt, R. W. Breast carcinoma. *Hum. Pathol.* 9:3, 1978.
30. McDivitt, R. W., Stewart, F. W., and Berg, J. W. *Tumors of the Breast: Atlas of Tumor Pathology* (Second Series, Fasc. 2). Washington, D.C.: Armed Forces Institute of Pathology, 1968.

31. Norris, H. J., and Taylor, H. B. Relationship of histologic features to behavior of cystosarcoma phyllodes. *Cancer* 20:2090, 1967.
32. Nussbaum, H., Kagan, A. R., Gilbert, H., et al. Management of inflammatory breast carcinoma. *Breast* 3:25, 1977.
33. Pietruszka, M., and Barnes, L. Cystosarcoma phyllodes. *Cancer* 41:1974, 1978.
34. Robbins, G. F., and Berg, J. W. Bilateral primary breast cancers. *Cancer* 17:1501, 1964.
35. Rosen, P. P., Fracchia, A. A., Urban, J. A., et al. "Residual" mammary carcinoma following simulated partial mastectomy. *Cancer* 35:739, 1975.
36. Rosen, P. P., Lieberman, P. H., Braun, D. W., et al. Lobular carcinoma in situ of the breast. Detailed analysis of 99 patients with average follow-up of 24 years. *Am. J. Surg. Pathol.* 2:225, 1978.
37. Rosen, P. P., Snyder, R. E., Urban, J., et al. Correlation of suspicious mammograms and x-rays of breast biopsies during surgery. Results in 60 cases. *Cancer* 31:656, 1973.
38. Saphir, O., and Amromin, G. D. Obscure axillary lymph node metastasis in carcinoma of the breast. *Cancer* 1:238, 1948.
39. Say, C. C., and Donegan, W. L. Invasive carcinoma of the breast: Prognostic significance of tumor size and involved axillary lymph nodes. *Cancer* 34:468, 1974.
40. Scheike, O., and Visfeldt, J. Male breast cancer: IV. Gynecomastia in patients with breast cancer. *Acta Pathol. Microbiol. Scand.* [A] 81:359, 1973.
41. Tsakraklides, V., Olson, P., Kersey, J. H., et al. Prognostic significance of the regional lymph node histology in cancer of the breast. *Cancer* 34:1259, 1974.
42. Urban, J. A., Papachristou, D., and Taylor, J. Bilateral breast cancer. Biopsy of the opposite breast. *Cancer* 40:1968, 1977.
43. Wheeler, J. E., and Enterline, H. T. Lobular carcinoma of the breast in situ and infiltrating. *Path. Annu.* 11:161, 1976.
44. Zajdela, A., Ghossein, N. A., Pilleron, J. P., et al. The value of aspiration cytology in the diagnosis of breast cancer: Experience at the Fondation Curie. *Cancer* 35:499, 1975.

Nelson A. Burstein

5. Biochemical Features of Breast Cancer

Interest in the biochemistry of breast cancer covers two areas: an understanding of the changes that occur in a cell as it undergoes malignant transformation, and the use of the biochemical properties of the tumor to select therapy for patients with breast cancer. This chapter focuses on the second, more practical, area. I consider the hormone receptor assays and discuss their methodology, uses, and limitations. In addition, certain other biochemical tests of tumor tissue that may predict response to chemotherapy are discussed. Finally, comments are included on the use of biomarkers in breast cancer patients.

Hormone Receptor Analysis

Currently, the most useful biochemical assay of the clinical hormone responsiveness of a breast carcinoma is the presence or absence of estrogen receptor (ER). This cytoplasmic protein has a high affinity for estradiol and is present in cells that are targets of estrogen action. The estrogen, usually estradiol, is thought to cross the cell membrane by passive diffusion and then bind to the receptor. Once the receptor has interacted with the estrogen, the protein undergoes a change in size or shape. This irreversibly altered receptor-estrogen complex can then enter the nucleus and bind to chromatin. As a result of this nuclear binding, the cell may synthesize DNA and proliferate. Alternately, the cell may produce RNA and appropriately differentiated products, such as receptors for other hormones and enzymes for differentiated function [18, 26]. The breast, as a target tissue for estrogen, would be expected to have a receptor for estrogen.

An understanding of the various assay methods used to measure the estrogen receptor is clinically relevant. The tumor sample is homogenized and then centrifuged to remove particulate matter. The soluble cytoplasmic fraction containing the receptor is incubated with radioactive estradiol both with and without a specific inhibitor of binding (usually diethylstilbestrol). The free and bound estradiol are separated and counted. The differences

Table 5-1   Estrogen Receptors in Breast Cancer

Age of Patients	Number of Patients Tested (total, 402)	% Patients Showing Positive Receptors*	Mean fm/mg Protein of Those Positive
0–30	16	50	9.4
31–40	39	46	16.0
41–50	95	53	23.1
51–60	106	59	40.4
61–70	80	73	51.8
71–80	48	75	60.8
80+	18	83	69.1

*3 fm/mg protein is the lower limit for positivity.

between the radioactivity in the tubes correspond to the specific binding, usually calculated and expressed in fentomoles (fm, 10–15 moles). In all assays some reference is made to the amount of tissue used, and this is usually expressed as milligrams of protein. Illustrated examples are found in Table 5–1. For convenience, the patients discussed are divided by age. Approximately half of the tumors from premenopausal patients are estrogen receptor positive. A higher percentage of positives occur in the postmenopausal group, and there is also an increase in the level of binding in the older patients. This is not merely owing to the presence of more available sites because of lower circulating estrogen, but represents some as yet unexplained feature of the tumor in older patients [23].

Table 5–2 summarizes a cooperative study evaluating clinical response to endocrine therapy in patients with estrogen receptor data [23]. Here we see that 43 to 60 percent of patients with estrogen receptor positive tumors will respond to some form of endocrine manipulation. Of those tumors without estrogen receptors, fewer than 10 percent respond to therapy. The exact form of therapy seems to make little difference to the correlation; for example, if a premenopausal patient responds to oophorectomy, the tumor will likely be estrogen receptor positive, and if a postmenopausal patient responds to estrogen, the tumor will be estrogen receptor positive. Responders to androgen also will be estrogen receptor positive. One can postulate and eventually test many hypotheses to ex-

Table 5-2. Objective Breast Tumor Regressions According to Estrogen Receptor (ER) Assay and Type of Therapy as Judged by Extramural Review [23]

Therapy	ER +	ER −	ER ±
Adrenalectomy	32/66	4/33	3/8
Castration	25/33	4/53	0/2
Hypophysectomy	2/8	0/8	—
Total	59/107 (55%)	8/94 (8%)	3/10 (30%)
Androgen	12/26	2/24	0/1
Estrogen	37/57	5/58	0/2
Glucocorticoid	2/2	—	—
Total	51/85 (60%)	7/82 (8%)	0/3 (0%)
Antiestrogens	8/20	5/27	—
Other	2/3	0/5	—
Total	10/23 (43%)	5/32 (16%)	—

plain these and other correlations. At present, however, it is best to think of the presence of the receptor as a convenient marker of biochemical differentiation of the tumor—a marker that correlates with the tumor's general sensitivity to manipulations of its hormone environment.

A high degree of concurrence of results (up to 90 percent) exists between estrogen receptor assays of sequential and of multiple biopsies of primary tumors and metastases from the same patient. Thus, the assay data are useful in managing a patient who develops metastatic disease several years later. There is no general correlation with histology of the tumor [23], although there may be a slight increase in receptor positivity in the group with lobular carcinoma [28]. Poorly differentiated tumors rarely contain estrogen receptor. There is no correlation between stage of disease and presence of receptor. However, there is some evidence that patients who were ER + will have metastases to bone more frequently than to the liver and conversely those who were ER − will more frequently have metastases to the liver [31]. There may be evidence that patients with a positive ER have a better prognosis [19].

Additional aspects of the estrogen receptor have been

studied to increase the predictive accuracy. Most laboratories have a threshold for positivity, usually 3 to 10 fm/mg protein. When one compares the amount of receptor with the probability of response, there are few responders below 3 fm/mg protein; on the other hand, over 80 percent of patients will respond when the level is over 100 fm/mg protein [14, 24].

In an attempt to increase the predictive value of the in-vitro tests, other receptors have been evaluated. Progesterone receptor (PR) has shown the most promise, and from a theoretical standpoint, this approach has appeal. The cytoplasmic progesterone receptor protein is synthesized by a target cell (e.g., breast or uterus) as a result of estrogen stimulation. Thus, if a cell contained progesterone receptor, the cell would not only have an estrogen receptor and be able to move that receptor to the nucleus, but it could also induce the production of progesterone receptor. This PR would serve as a marker of the completeness of estrogen sensitivity of the cell. Early reports [17] suggested the value of both ER assay and PR assay to predict response to endocrine manipulation. Notwithstanding the relative difficulty of this additional assay, it appears that there is only a slight increase in predictive value when both assays are used when compared with the use of the ER assay alone [24]. Moreover, the presence of PR positivity follows the level of ER; thus, a quantitative ER should and does give almost the same prediction. Finally, there is little evidence at present to exclude a patient from endocrine therapy if her tumor contains an ER but no PR.

Other receptors have been found in human breast cancer. These include androgen [36], glucocorticoid [33], insulin [27], and prolactin [5]. As with progesterone, there is a general correlation between the presence of these receptors and an increasing level of estrogen receptor. At present, there is little evidence of clinical application of these receptor assays.

The receptor assay has its greatest value in receptor negative tumors. Thus, the clinician should be aware of problems or errors that can produce a false negative laboratory test. The first common error is to test nontumorous tissue, which may include cavity walls with only granulation tissue or "skin recurrences" that contain only scar tissue. All samples should be malignant, and a histologic section should be taken from adjacent tissue for confirmation. Normal breast tissue adjacent to a tumor will not bind estrogen in the usual assay procedures. Samples that have been frozen in cryostat embedding medium and those containing too few cancer cells will also produce a false negative result. When our laboratory assays a very fibrous recurrence, bone biopsy, or effusion pellet, it lowers the cutoff level for positivity and cautions the clinician on the limited value of a negative assay. Inadequate freezing or chilling of the sample will lower the estrogen receptor content and produce false negative data.

The clinical false positive aspect of the assay deserves some mention. About 60 percent of all "positive" tumors respond to therapy. While this represents an improvement over the 20 to 30 percent of patients who usually respond to endocrine therapy, the predictability is still incomplete.

The tumors that do not respond to endocrine therapy despite hormone binding most likely represent a population of both hormone-dependent and hormone-independent cells. Perhaps this mixed population can be studied using the fluorescent-labeled antibody to estrogen receptor [20].

It should be remembered, too, that the individual positive cells may have a varying amount of receptor. The mixed population hypothesis is consistent with the clinical observations of transient, partial, and mixed responses of different metastases to therapy. Furthermore, tumor cells may have altered mechanisms of response to hormonal stimuli. For example, in one tumor cell line that is inhibited by the antiestrogen tomoxifen, the estrogen receptor is present in the nucleus interacting with the chromatin in the apparent absence of estrogen [40]. Other evidence suggests that the cytoplasmic receptor of some tumors cannot translocate to the nucleus or has an altered affinity or specificity for estradiol [21].

The theoretical aspects of hormone dependence are exciting. As new model systems are introduced, we learn of more ways in which hormonal information can be conveyed and confused in a tumor cell. These are interesting and may allow for the development of new drugs and hormones directed at these defects in individual patients. Today, however, the predictive value of the estrogen receptor assay is clear. If the assay is negative (usually below 3 fm/mg protein in a premenopausal patient or 7 to 10 fm/mg protein in a postmenopausal woman), the patient has less than a 10 percent chance of responding to endocrine therapy. If it is positive, then, depending on the level of receptor and other factors such as site of disease, length of disease-free interval, and so on, the patient has about a 60 percent chance of responding to some form of therapy that will alter the endocrine environment of the tumor.

The presence of estrogen receptor in a breast carcinoma may be related to factors other than hormone responsiveness. Earlier we noted that a greater proportion of tumors from postmenopausal women contain receptor. Some reports show that the presence of receptor is an independent variable in assessing prognosis [19]. There is an inverse relationship between receptor presence and mitotic index and growth rate [25]. Initial reports suggested that response of tumors to chemotherapy was associated with absence of estrogen receptor [22]. Subsequent studies show no such association [15].

Additional Biochemical Tumor Properties

Other biochemical properties of breast carcinoma may be of significance in therapy. The normal breast is capable of converting androgens to estrogens [1]. This property is retained in carcinomas that respond to adrenalectomy [6]. In contrast to the normal breast and in benign disease, carcinoma produces increased levels of glycolytic enzymes [16]. These differences are most notable in lactate dehydrogenase (LDH) and pyruvate kinase (PK). Significant increases are also seen in glucosephosphate isomerase (GPI), hexokinase, and phosphoglucomutase (PGM). Elevation of two other nonglycolytic enzymes, glucose-6-phosphate dehydrogenase and the NADP-isocitrate dehydrogenase (ICD), are also seen. Levels of these enzymes bear an inverse relationship with estrogen receptor [16] and, independently, an apparent relationship with response of the tumor to combination chemotherapy [29]. Initially, GPI, LDH, ICD, and PK showed the most promise as predictors. In subsequent analysis with more patients, it appears the LDH still predominates as a factor along with the ratio of the ICD/PGM. These levels, when expressed in the appropriate mathematical model, did predict a probability of response to chemotherapy in 32 of 37 patients [8].

Biomarkers of Breast Cancer

The ideal biomarker of breast cancer would permit early diagnosis in screened populations. Moreover, it would discriminate between patients who have had successful primary therapy and those with micrometastases. Finally, it would permit adequate monitoring of the tumor's response to therapy. Unfortunately, this ideal or even near-ideal marker does not exist. However, several biomarkers do exist in breast cancer patients that may be useful in clinical management.

Carcinoembryonic Antigen

Perhaps the most useful of biomarkers is the carcinoembryonic antigen (CEA). This glycoprotein was first noted in the serum and tumors of patients with colonic malignancies [11]. Further work demonstrated this antigen in patients with nongastrointestinal malignacies such as those in the breast, lung, and ovary [13]. In one series [3], over one half of women with primary breast cancer had an elevated CEA in contrast to approximately 10 percent of normal controls. In patients with metastatic disease, the CEA was elevated 70 percent of the time. In 22 patients with metastasis and elevated CEA, the level of CEA rose and fell directly with the clinical response of the tumor to therapy. Higher levels of CEA seemed to be associated with a worse prognosis. Elevated CEA levels were seen more frequently (over 70%) in patients with bone and liver involvement than in those with skin and breast involvement (50%) [35]. Although the test may have some value in screening populations for breast cancer, its greatest use is in following the patient who already has cancer. The fluctuation in CEA level with the growth and regression of the metastatic tumor is a sensitive indicator of response to therapy and early recurrence.

Human Chorionic Gonadotropin

The normal placental product, human chorionic gonadotropin (HCG), is present in about one half of patients with breast cancer [34]. HCG elevations were seen in 5 of 14 patients with operable disease and in 65 of 134 patients with metastatic disease. In the few patients with recurrent disease, 4 of 10 had preceding elevations of HCG. In patients with detectable HCG, the lower levels of HCG were associated with a greater response rate to chemotherapy (over 90 percent in those with less than 5 mIU/ml). There is evidence that the levels of HCG reflect tumor mass and may parallel the response of the tumor to therapy [34].

Another placental hormone, lactogen, is present in almost 20 percent of patients with primary breast cancer [30]. Here, however, its value for screening and following the course of the disease is unknown.

Possible Useful Biomarkers

In the following sections, I will comment on biomarkers that may eventually prove useful but are still limited in their clinical application. One such group is the protein-bound carbohydrates. Fucose appears to be the most useful. Elevations can be seen in the serum levels of patients with malignant breast lesions in contrast to levels in normal women or those with benign disease [32]. In some reports, the serum fucose to protein ratio was elevated in over 90 percent of patients with metastatic carcinomas [7]. In another report, a slightly lower incidence (85%) of elevated fucose was seen in 150 patients with metastatic breast carcinoma [37]. In these patients, the level fell during response to therapy and rose preceding obvious clinical recurrence.

A glycoprotein normally seen in pregnancy is also associated with breast cancer. When this pregnancy-associated alpha-macroglobulin was evaluated in 30 patients who went on to develop recurrent disease, all patients had a rise in this biomarker 1 to 21 months before clinical evidence of recurrence [2]. The baseline in this assay can vary from patient to patient; however, the elevation over time was a consistent feature for each patient with recurrence.

The levels of casein, a secretory product of the normal breast, tend to be elevated in patients with local and metastatic breast cancer. There is considerable overlap with normal patients, however [9]. Moreover, longitudinal studies are unavailable to evaluate its usefulness in following response to therapy.

A glycoprotein found in breast cyst fluid is another useful

marker for breast cancer. It is elevated most in those patients with metastatic disease and to a lesser degree in those with localized malignancy and gross cystic disease. There was a further suggestion that the level of this glycoprotein paralleled the change in tumor volume [12].

Hydroxyproline excretion is a useful marker for patients with metastatic breast cancer [10]. This urinary metabolite of collagen breakdown is elevated in bone metastasis and is helpful as an adjunct to the bone scan. Changes in the hydroxyproline/creatinine ratio may be useful in following the early response to therapy in metastatic disease.

Urinary levels of polyamines—namely spermidine, spermine, and putresine—are increased in patients with malignant disease [4]. This presumably is related to neoplastic growth. Urinary nucleosides are similarly elevated. These include pseudouridine, N^2N^2-dimethylguanosine and 1-methylinosine [38]. By themselves, these groups of markers are not as useful as CEA in predicting the presence of either metastatic disease or actual changes in tumor burden. Their predictive value is increased when the polyamine levels are considered with the nucleosides and the CEA [39].

In conclusion, a variety of biomarkers of malignancy are present in breast cancer. None is specific and unique to breast cancer. Some of the general markers, such as CEA and HCG, may be useful when following a patient for recurrence or response to therapy if the marker was originally present. Other, more specific, breast markers, such as casein and glycoproteins, may be present in the normal population. Urinary hydroxyproline may be helpful in diagnosing early bony metastases. Finally, urinary polyamines and nucleosides may prove useful markers, especially when combined with CEA.

References

1. Adams, J. B., and Wong, M. S. F. Paraendocrine behaviour of human breast carcinoma. In vitro transformation of steroids to physiologically active hormones. *J. Endocrinol.* 41:41, 1968.
2. Anderson, M., Stimson, W. H., and Kelly, F. Preclinical warning of recrudescent mammary cancers by pregnancy-associated alpha-macroglobulin. *Br. J. Surg.* 63:819, 1976.
3. Borthwick, N. M., Wilson, D. W., and Bell, P. A. Carcinoembryonic antigen (CEA) in patients with breast cancer. *Eur. J. Cancer* 13:171, 1977.

4. Cohen, S. S. (Chairman). Meeting report: Conference on polyamines in cancer. *Cancer Res.* 37:939, 1977.
5. Cole, E. N., Golder, M. P., and Griffiths, K. Prolactin in human breast tumours. *Proc. Soc. Endocrinol.* 49P, 1975.
6. Dao, T. L., and Libby, P. R. Conjugation of hormones by breast cancer tissue and selection of patients for adrenalectomy. *Surgery* 66:162, 1969.
7. Evans, A. S., Dolan, M. F., Sobocinski, P. X., et al. Utility of serum protein-bound neutral hexoses and L-fucose for estimation of malignant tumor extension and evaluation of efficacy of therapy. *Cancer Res.* 34:538, 1974.
8. Feldstein, M. L., Savlov, E. D., and Hilf, R. A statistical model for predicting response of breast cancer patients to cytotoxic chemotherapy. *Cancer Res.* 38:2544, 1978.
9. Franchimont, P., and Zangerle, P. F. Present and future clinical relevance of tumour markers. *Eur. J. Cancer* 13:637, 1971.
10. Gielen, F., Dequeker, J., Drochmans, A., et al. Relevance of hydroxyproline excretion to bone metastasis in breast cancer. *Br. J. Cancer* 34:279, 1976.
11. Gold, P., and Freedman, S. O. Demonstration of tumour-specific antigens in human colonic carcinomata by immunologic tolerance and absorption techniques. *J. Exp. Med.* 121:439, 1965.
12. Haagensen, D. E., Mazoujian, G., Holder, W. D., et al. Evaluation of a breast cyst fluid protein detectable in the plasma of breast carcinoma patients. *Ann. Surg.* 185:279, 1977.
13. Hansen, H. J., Snyder, J. J., Miller, E., et al. CEA assay: A laboratory adjunct in the diagnosis and management of cancer. *Human Pathol.* 5:139, 1974.
14. Heuson, J. C., Longeval, E., Mattheiem, W. H., et al. Significance of quantitative assessment of estrogen receptors for endocrine therapy in advanced breast cancer. *Cancer* 39:1971, 1977.
15. Hilf, R., Feldstein, M. L., Gibson, S. L., et al. The relative importance of estrogen receptor analysis as a prognostic factor for recurrence or response to chemotherapy in women with breast cancer. *Cancer* 45:1993, 1980.
16. Hilf, R., and Wittliff, J. L. Characterization of Human Breast Cancer by Examination of Cytoplasmic Enzyme Activities and Estrogen Receptors. In K. W. McKerns (Ed.), *Hormones and Cancer.* New York: Academic, 1974.
17. Horwitz, K. B., McGuire, W. L., Pearson, O. H., et al. A predicting response to endocrine therapy in human breast cancer: A hypothesis. *Science* 189:726, 1975.
18. Jensen, E. V., and DeSombre, E. R. Estrogen-receptor interaction. *Science* 182:126, 1973.
19. Knight, W. A., Livingston, R. B., Gregory, E. J., et al. Estrogen receptor as an independent prognostic factor for early recurrence in breast cancer. *Cancer Res.* 37:4669, 1977.
20. Lee, S. H. Cytochemical study of estrogen receptor in human mammary cancer. *Am. J. Clin. Pathol.* 70:197, 1978.

21. Lippman, M. E., and Allegra, J. C. Current concepts in cancer: Receptors in breast cancer. Estrogen receptor and endocrine therapy of breast cancer. *N. Engl. J. Med.* 299:930, 1978.

22. Lippman, M. E., Allegra, J. C., Thompson, E. B., et al. The relation between estrogen receptors and response rate to cytotoxic chemotherapy in metastatic breast cancer. *N. Engl. J. Med.* 298:1223, 1978.

23. McGuire, W. L., Carbone, P. P., and Vollmer, E. P. (Eds.). *Estrogen Receptors in Human Breast Cancer.* New York: Raven Press, 1975.

24. McGuire, W. L., Zava, D. T., Horwitz, K. B., et al. Receptors and breast cancer; do we know it all? *J. Steroid Biochem.* 9:461, 1978.

25. Meyer, J. S., Rao, B. R., Stevens, S. C., et al. Low incidence of estrogen receptor in breast carcinomas with rapid rates of cellular replication. *Cancer* 40:2290, 1977.

26. O'Malley, B. W., and Means, A. R. Female steroid hormones and target cell nuclei. *Science* 183:610, 1974.

27. Osborne, C. K., Monaco, M. E., Lippman, M. D., et al. Correlation among insulin binding, degradation, and biological activity in human breast cancer cells in long-term tissue culture. *Cancer Res.* 38:94, 1978.

28. Rosen, P. P., Menendez-Botet, C. J., Nisselbaum, J. S., et al. Pathological review of breast lesions analyzed for estrogen receptor protein. *Cancer Res.* 35:3187, 1975.

29. Savlov, E. D., Wittliff, J. L., Hilf, R., et al. Correlations between certain biochemical properties of breast cancer and response to therapy: A preliminary report. *Cancer* 33:303, 1974.

30. Sheth, N. A., Suraiya, J. N., Sheth, A. R., et al. Ectopic production of human placental lactogen by human breast tumors. *Cancer* 39:1693, 1977.

31. Singhakowinta, A., Potter, H. G., Buroker, T. R., et al. Estrogen receptor and natural course of breast cancer. *Ann. Surg.* 183:34, 1976.

32. Tatsumura, T., Sato, H., Mori, A., et al. Clinical significance of fucose level in glycoprotein fraction of serum in patients with malignant tumors. *Cancer Res.* 37:4101, 1977.

33. Teulings, F. A. G., and van Gilse, H. A. Demonstration of glucocorticoid receptors in human mammary carcinomas. *Hormone Res.* 8:107, 1977.

34. Tormey, D. C., Waalkes, T. P., and Simon, R. M. Biological markers in breast carcinoma: II. Clinical correlations with human chorionic gonadotrophin. *Cancer* 39:2391, 1977.

35. Tormey, D. C., Waalkes, T. P., Snyder, J. J., et al. Biological markers in breast carcinoma: III. Clinical correlations with carcinoembryonic antigen. *Cancer* 39:2397, 1977.

36. Trams, G., and Mass, H. Specific binding of estradiol and dihydrotestosterone in human mammary carcinomas. *Cancer Res.* 37:258, 1977.

37. Waalkes, T. P., Gehrke, C. W., Tormey, D. C., et al. Biological markers in breast carcinoma: IV. Serum fucose-protein ratio. Comparisons with carcinoembryonic antigen and human chorionic gonadotrophin. *Cancer* 41:1871, 1978.
38. Waalkes, T. P., Gehrke, C. M., Zumwalt, R. W., et al. The urinary excretion of nucleosides of ribonucleic acid by patients with advanced cancer. *Cancer* 36:390, 1975.
39. Woo, K. B., Waalkes, T. P., Ahmann, D. L., et al. A quantitative approach to determining disease response during therapy using multiple biologic markers. *Cancer* 41:1685, 1978.
40. Zava, D. T., and McGuire, W. L. Estrogen receptor. Unoccupied sites in nuclei of a breast tumor cell line. *J. Biol. Chem.* 252:3703, 1977.

Carl J. D'Orsi
Edward H. Smith

6. Breast Imaging

Mammography

Mammography, or soft tissue roentgenography of the breast, is not a new procedure. As early as 1913 Salomon [56] used roentgenography to study gross pathologic breast specimens. Clinical application lagged behind, however, and Warren [63] is generally credited with introducing mammography as a potentially important diagnostic tool; in 1930 he reported on 119 cases, 58 of which were malignant. Reports concerning mammography then began to appear in the medical literature, but enthusiasm was not great, mainly because the technical quality of the examinations was poor. In the early 1950s the technique began to attract wider clinical interest, and this interest must be ascribed to the work of Leborgne [39, 40]. He introduced the principles of low voltage accompanied by compression of the breast with which specialized x-ray film and cassettes were utilized; he also demonstrated calcification in malignancies and categorized some of the criteria used in the diagnosis of benign and malignant disease [39]. The evolving awareness of mammography as a clinically useful technique was further enhanced by Ingleby and Gershon-Cohen [27], who made extensive correlations between breast sections and their radiographs. In 1960 Egan [13] evaluated 1000 mammograms and provided the first satisfactory statistical analysis of consecutive mammograms in the American literature. A further refinement in technique was brought about by the use of xeroradiography, pioneered by Wolfe and associates [66, 68].

Technique and Imaging

Mammography requires excellent delineation of minute structures, not only for characterizing lesions but also for examining surrounding structures in the breast. In general, low-peak kilovoltage (KV) coupled with adequate milliamps is necessary to secure sufficient exposure at the lower KV. If film is to be used rather than xerography, strict adherence to collimation with a short object-film distance should be practiced.

The mammographic examination routinely includes two views of each breast, a craniocaudal and a mediolateral view. With both views breast tissue must be compressed in order to minimize exposure and increase radiographic detail of the breast tissue. Various techniques for compressing breast tissue have been developed, ranging from a balloon fitted into the radiographic cone to a movable plastic shield.

The two recording systems in use today are film and xeroradiographic processing. The industrial-type film with a fine grain that was initially used produced excellent radiographic detail. However, as will be discussed in the next section, the dose to the breast was large, and a search for better film-screen combinations was undertaken. Xeroradiography was first used as an alternate means of recording images in the early 1970s, largely because of the pioneering work of Dr. John Wolfe. This method involves the production of an electrostatic image that is then coated with powder, placed on paper, and finally coated with plastic (Fig. 6–1).

There are several advantages to using this technique for mammography. The most important is the "edge enhancement" effect. Xeroradiography tends to accentuate margins between areas of different radiographic density more than would ordinarily be expected, enabling better analysis of the edge characteristics of mass lesions. The dose is also lower than that required for industrial-type film. A greater latitude of recording is obtained, allowing visualization of good soft tissue detail as well as calcific or osseous detail with one set of exposure factors. This becomes important when dealing with the large breast with fibrocystic disease. Resolution, at least in vitro [47], is said to be increased over film recording devices. Subjectively the examinations are easier to read; a view box is not required and reader fatigue is diminished.

Recently, in response to increased concern with induction of breast carcinoma by x-ray coupled with screening of asymptomatic women, the so-called low-dose systems have evolved. By reintroducing a screen-film combination with a vacuum inside the film cassette to ensure optimal film-screen contact, a further reduction in dose has occurred without much sacrifice in image quality.

In summary, the techniques currently in use for mammography include xeroradiography and several low-dose systems

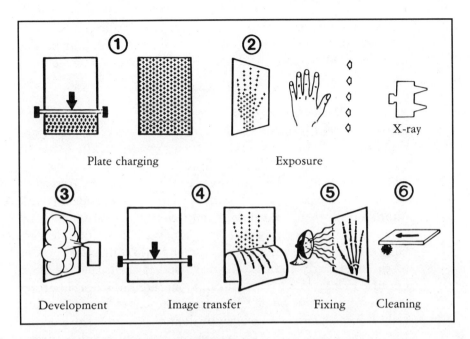

Figure 6–1. Xerographic process.

that use compression of the breast and views in the craniocaudal and mediolateral projections. With whatever method, both breasts must be examined even though the clinical area of suspicion is limited to one breast.

Screening, Dosimetry, and Carcinogenic Risk

According to estimates of the American Cancer Society, approximately 90,000 new cases of breast cancer will be detected each year and 33,000 deaths will result annually from the disease, making it the largest single cause of death in American women. If we accept that early diagnosis is correlated with improved survival, we can only improve the dismal statistics by some form of screening. Screening may be used for referring large numbers of asymptomatic women for examination in order to discover early tumors. As discussed in an earlier chapter, because risk factors for breast carcinoma are known, a subgroup (women known to be at risk) within the larger group of clinically asymptomatic women can be defined and concentrated on. Ideally the method used for screening should be rapid, accurate, and safe for the patients on whom it is used.

Several methods are available as possible screening tools. The first is the clinical examination by a physician who deals with diseases of the breast. However, it is generally accepted that the primary lesion must reach approximately 1 cm in diameter before it can be palpated even by the experienced examiner [43]. Thermography, another method and one to be dealt with subsequently, is basically nonspecific. Ultrasound holds promise, but much work still must be done before its accuracy makes it useful as a screening tool. Mammography, and specifically xeroradiography, fulfils many of the criteria for an ideal screening tool. It is a rapid examination and is safe for the patient. It has an approximately 85 percent true positive rate for diagnosing malignant disease [68], and lesions as small as 1 to 2 mm can be detected.

The assumption of improved survival secondary to earlier diagnosis of breast cancer coupled with the high accuracy and relative ease of performance of mammography led to the institution of several large breast-cancer screening programs, the most widely publicized being the Health Insurance Plan (HIP) study of New York.

The HIP study [57, 58] represented two systematic random

samples, each of which contained 31,000 women from 40 to 64 years of age. Women in the study group were offered a screening mammogram and three additional examinations at annual intervals, while women in the control group followed their usual practice in receiving medical care. In the study group 60 percent had all four examinations, 28 percent had two or three examinations, and 12 percent had only the first examination. Over the 7-year period of the study, there were 70 deaths due to breast cancer in the study group as compared with 108 in the control group, which is statistically significant. The largest difference between the control group and the study group was found in women in the 50-years-and-up age bracket, with almost no differences observed under 50 years of age. Similar statistics were obtained from the twenty-seven Breast Cancer Detection Demonstration Programs of the National Cancer Institute (NCI).

One of the considerations in any screening examination, or for that matter, any medical procedure, is to ensure that the procedure itself is not harmful. In the mid-1970s, considerable doubt was cast on the safety of mammography, particularly when examinations were repeated at various intervals. Bailar [3–5] felt that data was lacking on the long-term effects of dose on breast tissue from mammography and that the possible benefits of mammography had received more emphasis than its risks.

The dose to the breast is measured at the skin surface and varies with the method used. Original film mammography recorded on industrial film produced a range of exposure from 2.8 to 7.2 rads (rads being a measure of absorbed radiation energy), with an average of 4.8 rads per exposure; routine mammography used two exposures per breast. For comparison purposes the routine chest film will average 30 millirads (mr) or 0.003 rads. With modifications, the modern xerography dose to the breast can be reduced to about 0.4 rads per exposure. The new low-dose systems are in the range of 0.2 to 0.3 rads per exposure.

Our current knowledge about induced breast cancer in women comes from three major patient sources: atomic bomb survivors [46, 62], women treated with x-rays for acute postpartum mastitis [59], and women who have had repeated fluoroscopic examinations of the chest [6]. Of 5200 women exposed to an approximate dose of 0 to 90 rads from the atomic bomb, 10 cases of carcinoma were discovered, with the expected number for unexposed women being 12.3 cases. Of women exposed to 790 rads, 11 cases were found in 1643 women; 4.3 cases would be expected if there was no exposure.

Age at exposure also was a factor in the development of breast cancer. For females who were exposed to 100 or more rads between the ages of 10 and 34, 23 of 1935 women were found to eventually have breast cancer, with the expected number being 5.2. Of those exposed when 35 to 50+ years of age, 11 cases of breast carcinoma in 994 women were subsequently discovered, with only 4.4 expected. This suggests that breast tissue of adolescent females may be more sensitive to radiation than that of older women. Of 571 women treated for postpartum mastitis with a mean dose of 247 rads, the relative risk of breast cancer was 3.2 over 20 to 34 years postradiation. Similarly, 41 observed versus 23 expected breast cancers occurred in patients with repeated fluoroscopies to the chest, whereas no excess (15 observed, 14.1 expected) was apparent among the comparison population. Of interest was the fact that no excess carcinoma occurred in patients who received between 1 and 99 rads at fluoroscopy.

When considering the problem of dose during mammographic screening and possible inducement of carcinoma, many factors must be appreciated. The term *screening* refers to completely asymptomatic women who are not at high risk. Women not in this category have some indication for mammography, and for these women the benefit would outweigh the risk. In analyzing the data of dose versus possible inducement of mammary carcinoma, it should be noted that much of the breast dose was estimated, and the risk appeared greatest and was roughly linearly related to doses over 100 rads. Little or no factual information on doses in the mammographic range exist.

This problem is further compounded by current methods of measuring exposure during mammography. Previous estimates have included a rule of thumb that states that the dose at the midbreast in rads should be equal to 0.25 × surface exposure. This is inaccurate. Recently the midbreast dose exposure has been shown to be four times less than previously postulated for xeromammography and up to twenty times less with low-dose film mammography [20]. The final and most relevant question to be answered is, "Will the screening be worth the risk?" There appears to be evidence that the benefit does outweigh the risk

[48]. Using standard statistical techniques in the HIP study, a saving of 25 to 27 lives per 20,000 women screened was found. These lives were saved by mammography alone.

In summary, we recognize the theoretical risk of inducing carcinomas in a screened population, but we also realize the need to detect breast cancer earlier using modern equipment and recording systems that have reduced doses to acceptable levels. The guidelines set up by the American College of Radiology and the National Cancer Institute appear to represent a sensible approach [7, 61]. In asymptomatic women, the first or baseline mammographic examination should be performed between the ages of 35 and 40. Routine full screening of women under 50 years of age should probably be discontinued. In women over 50, annual or other regular interval examinations, including mammography, should be performed. The dose delivered should be kept as low as possible, and with current techniques should not exceed 1 rad to the midpoint of the breast per complete examination (two views).

Mass Lesions

For purposes of convenience, the signs seen on mammography can be divided into primary and secondary signs. The primary signs are those relating specifically to the mass itself, while secondary signs are those that occur because of what the malignant mass does to the surrounding breast.

Primary Signs. The primary signs as they relate to a mass are the shape and borders, density, and size of the lesion. The classic edge of the malignant mass is irregular or spiculate in nature (Fig. 6–2). On mammography the edge may present as a relatively smooth one with a hazy border (Fig. 6–3) or with numerous fine projections infiltrating the surrounding breast tissue. Larger projections, which give a stellate appearance to the mass and actually represent tumor filling the duct from the mass itself (Fig. 6–4) [14], may also be appreciated. Increased collagen deposition and distortion of surrounding ducts also add to the irregular shape and border of the mass [17].

The density of the tumor can be related to malignancy. Often these tumors are centrally dense. This has variously been attributed to more complete tumor replacement of normal breast tissue centrally [14] or to fibrosis or hemosiderin deposition, or both. The correlation of mammographic and clinical size of a breast mass is important in differentiating a benign lesion from

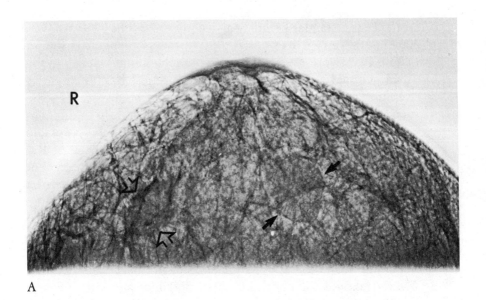

A

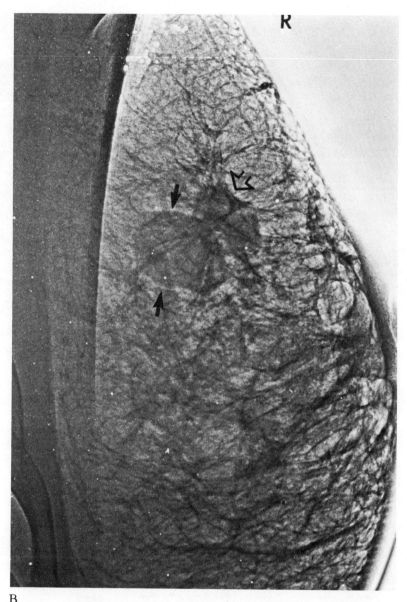

B

Figure 6–2. Malignant and benign masses. A. Craniocaudal xerogram showing smooth-bordered benign mass (*solid arrows*) adjacent
to more irregular malignant mass (*open arrows*). B. Lateral xerogram
showing malignant mass (*open arrow*) superimposed over benign
mass (*solid arrows*).

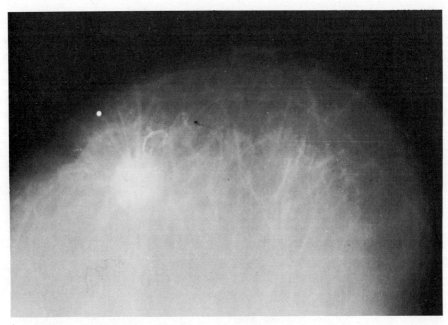

A

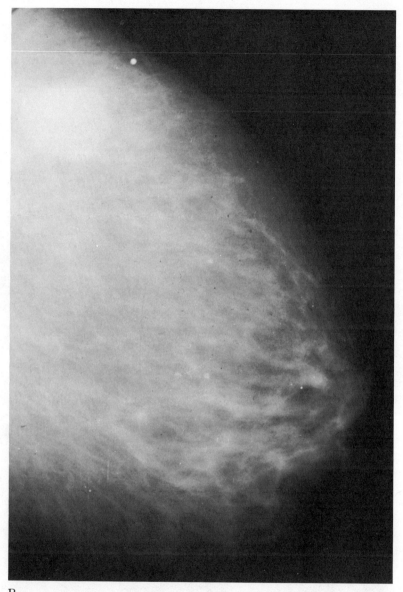

B
Figure 6–3. Film mammogram of a carcinoma. A. Craniocaudal view
of mass with hazy margins. B. Lateral view of same lesion.

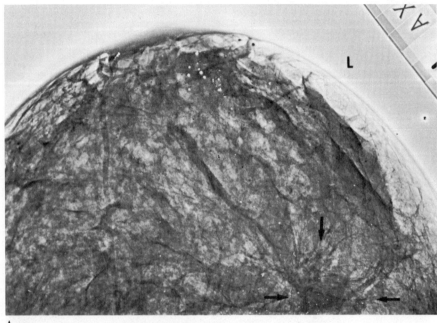

A

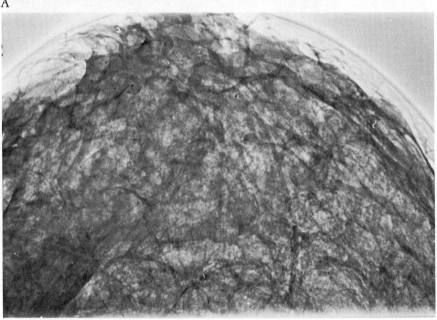

B

Figure 6-4. Stellate carcinoma. A. Craniocaudal view of stellate mass (*arrows*). The major radiographic component is its projections. B. View of contralateral side for comparison.

a malignant mass. The palpable mass may be two to four times the mammographic size. It is theorized that in this case the clinician is palpating the malignant mass and surrounding desmoplastic reaction, while mammography will usually only clearly visualize the dense malignant mass.

There are features of malignancy on mammography that cannot be categorized as either masses or suspicious calcifications. At times, malignancy may be first seen as an asymmetric area in the breast in comparison with the contralateral side (Fig. 6–5). Only major deviations from symmetry should be explored, although close clinical and radiographic follow-up of the patient is suggested for minor deviations. Carcinoma infiltrating duct tissue may not produce a discernible radiographic mass but will incite collagen formation in the periductal tissues. This is seen on mammography as a prominent duct pattern (Fig. 6–6). This assumes great importance as a sign for malignancy when it is only unilateral. Bilateral prominent ducts are a frequent finding in fibrocystic disease of the breast. The finding of a loss of the retromammary fat stripe unilaterally is ominous. Malignancy close to the retromammary fat may infiltrate it locally and obliterate an adjacent portion, even though it does not clearly present as a mass on mammograms.

Calcifications and Secondary Signs of Malignancy. The significance of calcifications in the breast (which can be found in both benign and malignant disease) has been recognized for many years [17]. Calcifications may be present in up to 75 percent of pathologically examined malignancies [33]. They assume importance when studying the breast radiographically, for they may provide the only evidence of malignancy.

Initially, the distinction between benign and malignant forms of calcification was felt to be rather clear-cut. Benign calcifications were large (1 mm and up), geometric, less numerous, and more uniformly distributed (Fig. 6–7); while the malignant variety were irregular, smaller (0.1–0.5 mm), and more clustered (Fig. 6–8). In general, this is true; for example, Rogers and Powell [53] found the presence of small (less than 0.3 mm) grouped calcifications to be the most frequent sign of a nonpalable malignancy. However, Millis [47] has demonstrated that the radiographic differentiation between benign and malignant calcifications is not as striking as was formerly believed.

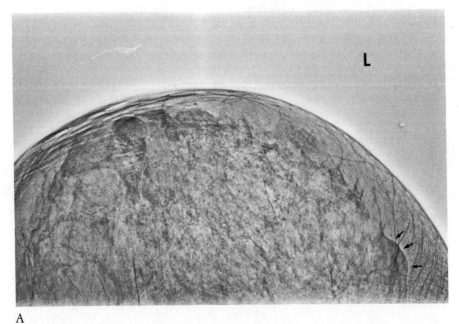

A

Figure 6–5. Asymmetric malignant density. Craniocaudal (A) and lateral (B) xerograms of bulging region in the upper outer quadrant (*arrows*).

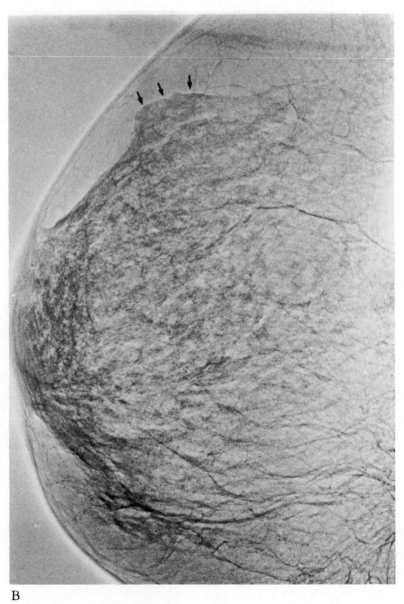

B

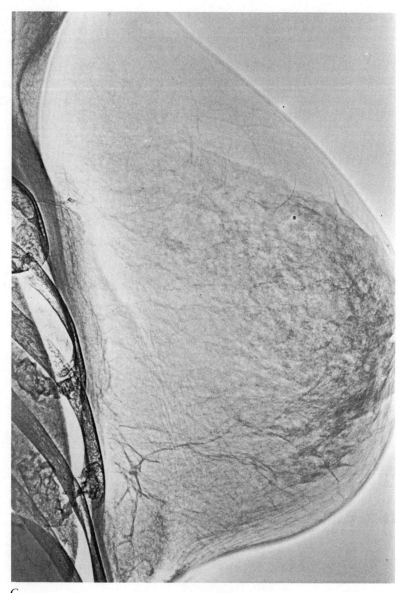

C
Figure 6–5 (Continued) Lateral view of the contralateral side does
not have a similar appearance.

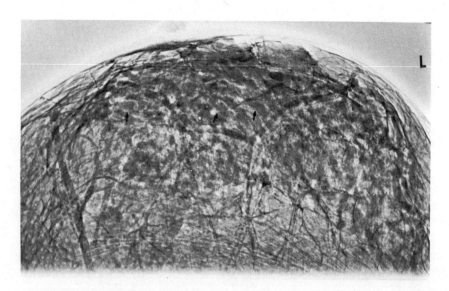

Figure 6–6. Prominent ducts. Small, oval, beaded densities (*arrows*) most prominent in the subareolar areas are typical for ducts and surrounding collagenosis.

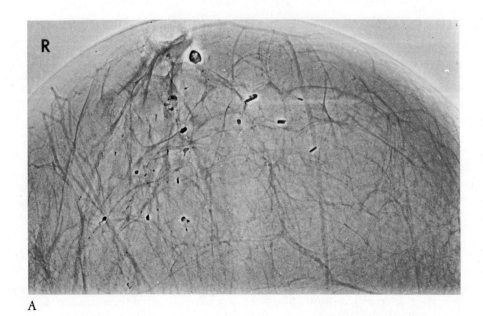

A

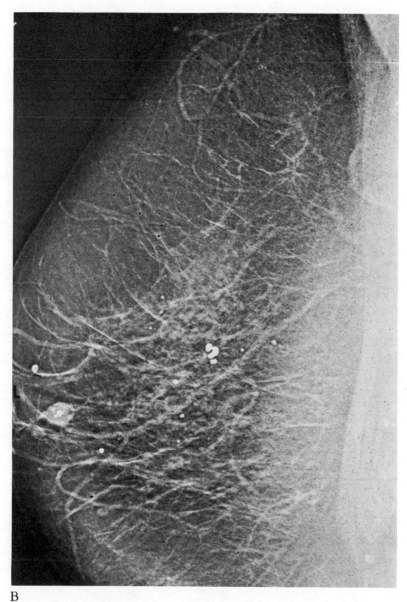

B

Figure 6–7. Benign calcification. A. One form of benign calcification, tubular and coarse in nature, representing ductal calcification. B. Lateral view with coarse ductal calcification widely spread throughout the glandular tissue. (Note reversal of technique so that calcium now appears white.)

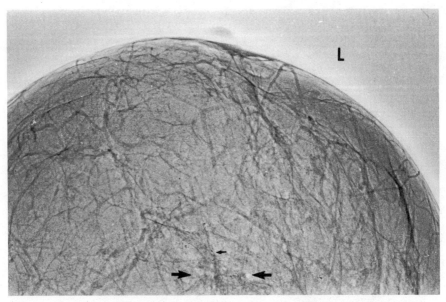

A

Figure 6–8. Malignant calcification. Ill-defined mass (*large arrows*) on craniocaudal (A) and lateral (B) views associated with small, punctate, clumped calcifications (*small arrows*).

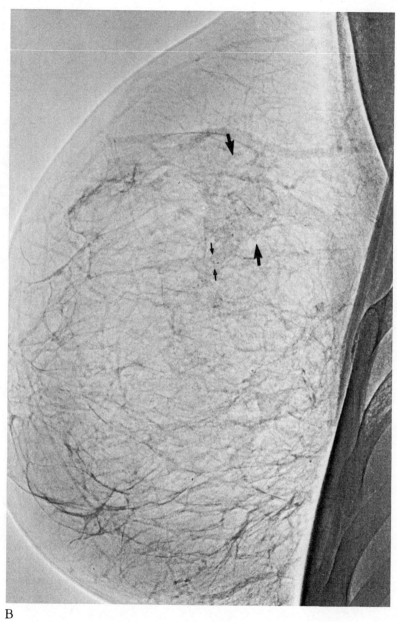

B

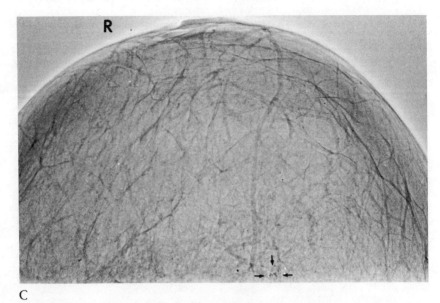

C

Figure 6–8 (Continued) C. Clumped calcifications unassociated with a mass lesion (*arrows*). D. Rather coarse but clumped calcifications (*open arrow*) associated with an ill-defined mass typical of malignancy (*large closed arrow*). Note benign ductal calcification (*small closed arrows*).

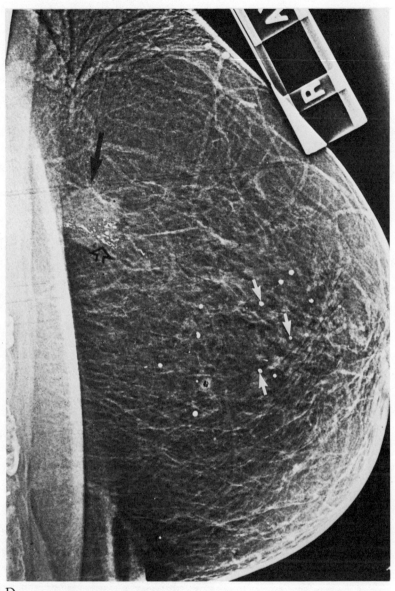

D

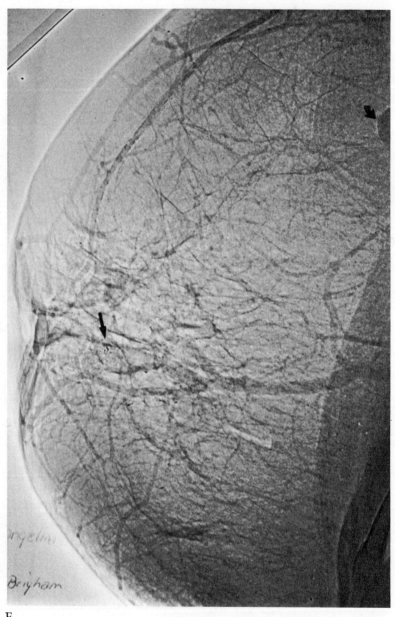

E

Figure 6–8 (Continued) E. Small area of calcification (*straight arrow*) with associated adenopathy (*curved arrow*). Biopsy revealed intraductal carcinoma.

Malignancies with coarse calcifications were encountered, and, conversely, benign diseases with fine, clumped calcifications were demonstrated. However, clustering and irregular shape appear to remain fairly important differential points.

In summary, the presence of calcifications assumes great importance in early detection of malignancy. Any cluster of calcifications, regardless of size—especially if they are irregular in shape and are not found on the contralateral side—should be biopsied. Calcifications that are borderline, that is, lacking tight clustering or having more regular shapes and appearing in both breasts, may be reexamined in six months to a year for changes in their appearance.

Secondary signs of malignancy include skin thickening, nipple or skin retraction, or both, and venous enlargement on one side only. In general, these findings are less meaningful when detected as isolated events but may be of significant aid in differentiating between benign and malignant mass lesions. The most important of these is skin thickening. Normally the skin over the breast measures about 1.5 mm (Fig. 6–9), except in the areolar area where it is thicker. A localized region of skin thickening becomes suspicious for an underlying malignancy. A careful search of the radiograph should be instituted when this is discovered (Fig. 6–10). The explanation offered for the thickening is an increase in collagen or dermal lymphatic obstruction, or both [17].

A secondary finding of equal importance is retraction of the skin and nipple, and indeed this almost always occurs in concert with skin thickening (Fig. 6–11). The desmoplastic response of malignant tumor, with its associated retractile property, is the most likely cause of retraction. One other point about nipple retraction should be emphasized. In many women inverted nipples are a normal finding; it is the onset of recent nipple inversion that is of more importance.

Other nonmalignant conditions may produce skin thickening. Fat necrosis and breast abscess will produce thickened skin. The postradiated breast will produce a generalized thickening as well. Usually a combination of clinical and radiographic findings will separate the benign from suspicious skin thickening.

The vascular pattern of the breast is surprisingly symmetric. When venous structures in similar quadrants of each breast were

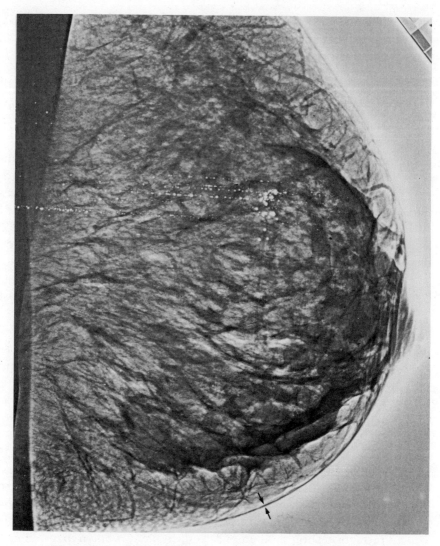

Figure 6–9. Normal skin. Lateral xerogram depicting normal breast skin thickness (*arrows*).

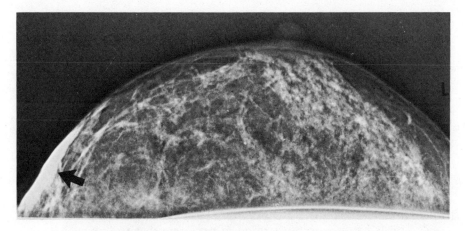

Figure 6–10. Abnormal skin thickness. Localized area of skin thickening (*arrow*) adjacent to small carcinoma.

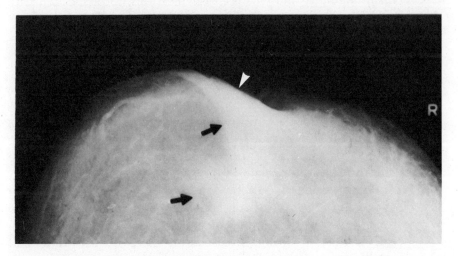

Figure 6–11. Malignant skin thickening and retraction. Film mammogram with constellation of mass and skin thickening (*arrows*) and nipple retraction from associated desmoplastic reaction (*arrowhead*).

measured, ratios of 1.4:1 or greater were found in a large percentage of patients with malignancy [11]. Unfortunately, several benign diseases, including fibrocystic disease, may produce the same finding. Thus, this particular secondary sign is the least specific and should only assume importance if it is found with one or more of the primary signs of malignancy (Fig. 6–12).

Lesion Localization and Specimen Radiography
The increased use of mammography for both screening and diagnosis has created problems when occult lesions have been demonstrated. Often, locating these lesions at operation has been extremely difficult; and wide excisions or quadrant resections have been performed in the hope that the suspicious area will be included in the excised tissue. The technique of localization, is specifically suited for nonpalpable masses seen on mammography and clustered calcifications not associated with palpable masses.

Localization allows the surgeon to visualize the lesion so the suspicious area can be excised. Toward this end one may use a 22-gauge needle (Fig. 6–13) or a variation thereof to locate the lesion within the breast [10, 16, 23, 41, 54]. Alternatively, a mixture of radiographic contrast and vital stain, such as methylene blue, may be injected in the area of suspicion. In this manner the lesion may be marked both radiographically for the radiologist and visually for the surgeon. In addition, a needle does not have to remain in the breast as a marker. The localization procedure should be done as close to the time of biopsy as possible, no more than 2 to 3 hours elapsing between the two. This becomes important when methylene blue is used, since diffusion through breast tissue increases with time, and marking specificity will be lost. After prior mammograms are reviewed, markers are placed on the craniocaudal and lateral surfaces of the breast at the levels of the lesion as judged by the mammogram. Craniocaudal and lateral views are then taken (Fig. 6–14). From these views, fairly accurate measurements of the lesion can be made.

Once the dimensions have been determined, the craniocaudal or lateral skin surface closest to the lesion is prepared. If one of the various needle localizations is to be used (see Fig. 6–13), the needle is inserted to the proper depth and repeat cranio-

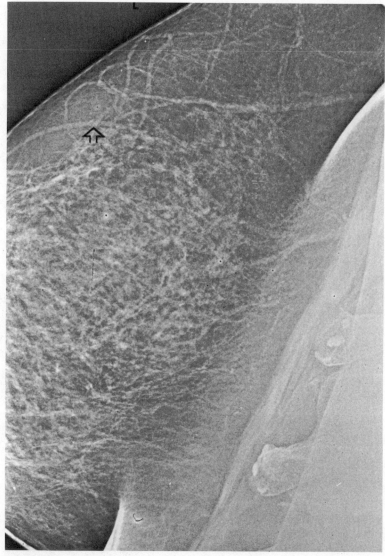

A

Figure 6–12. Venous asymmetry. A. Vein in upper half of breast (*open arrow*).

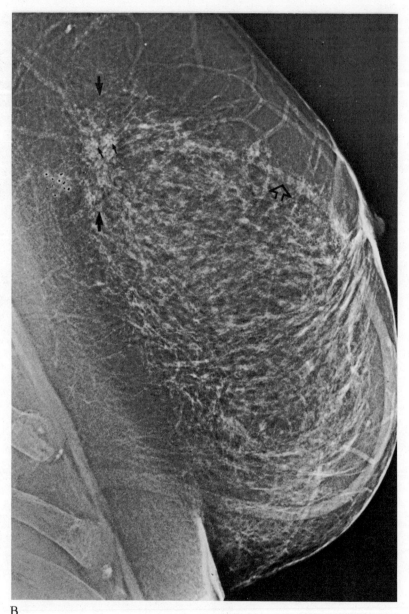

B

Figure 6–12 (Continued) B. Contralateral side shows increased venous diameter (*open arrow*) associated with malignant mass (*large arrows*) and calcification (*small arrows*).

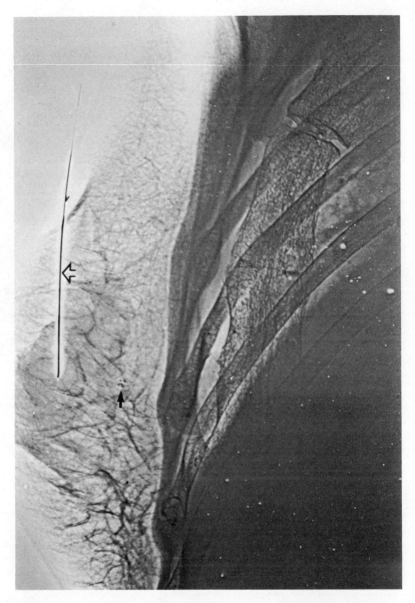

Figure 6–13. Needle method of localization. A 25-gauge needle (*open arrow*) is seen, the tip of which is just anterior to clumped malignant calcification (*solid arrow*).

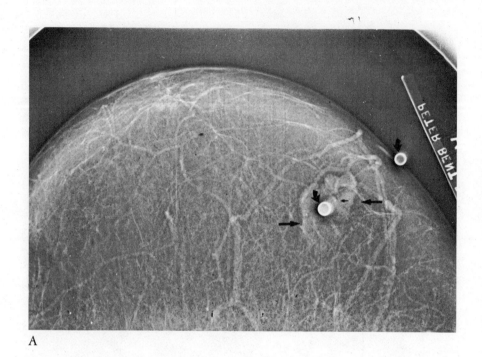

A

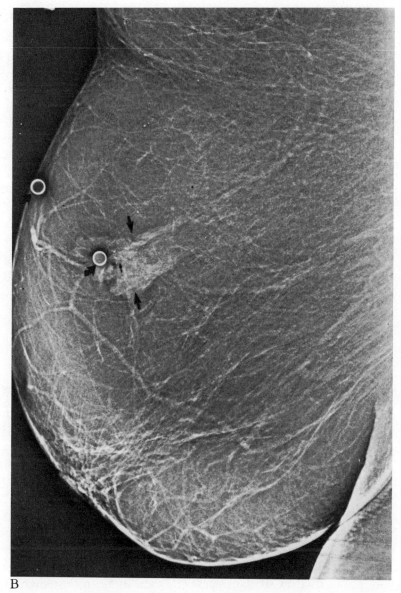

B

Figure 6–14. Lesion localization mammograms. Craniocaudal (A) and lateral (B) mammograms with metallic markers (*curved arrows*) adjacent to malignant mass (*straight arrows*) and malignant calcification (*small arrow*).

caudal and lateral views are done. If the marker is reasonably close to the lesion, measurements from the lesion are written on the film that is sent to the operating room with the patient. However, if a gross discrepancy is present, the needle may be reinserted and another set of films done. When a mixture of Renografin 60 and methylene blue is used for contrast, 0.5 ml of each are drawn up into a 3-ml syringe. A 25-gauge needle with a removable core is then inserted into the breast as for needle localization; at this time adjacency of the needle to the lesion may be confirmed by additional films. Approximately 0.3 ml of the mixture is introduced. Continuous injection is maintained as the needle is removed so that a fine linear track is produced. Postlocalization mammograms are then obtained (Fig. 6–15).

When the specimen has been removed it is radiographed, although this is usually done only for suspicious calcifications. Nonpalpable masses often may be distorted in excised tissue and may be difficult to differentiate. A small needle is placed in the area of suspicion and sent to pathology for frozen section (Fig. 6–16).

Mammographic Risk Patterns

It would be of obvious benefit, for both the screening of patients and for increasing cancer detection, if variations in breast parenchyma could be linked to degrees of carcinoma risk. Wolfe [67] has shown such an association in a retrospective analysis of 7214 patients. The classification is based on relative amounts of fat and glandular elements shown on the mammogram. The categories proceed from parenchyma composed primarily of fat (N1) to severe involvement with dysplasia or fibrocystic disease (DY). A parenchymal pattern made up primarily of fat but with prominent ducts up to one quarter of the volume of the breast (P1) and a severe prominent duct pattern involving more than one quarter of the breast (P2) are in an intermediate position (Fig. 6–17). Malignancy appears to be more prevalent in breasts assigned to the P2 and DY categories versus breasts with N1 and P1 classifications. Thus a gross estimate of risk for developing breast cancer can be assigned on the basis of breast parenchymal patterns. Although some doubt has been cast on the absolute percentage of risk for each category [44], the general trend appears to be significant [19].

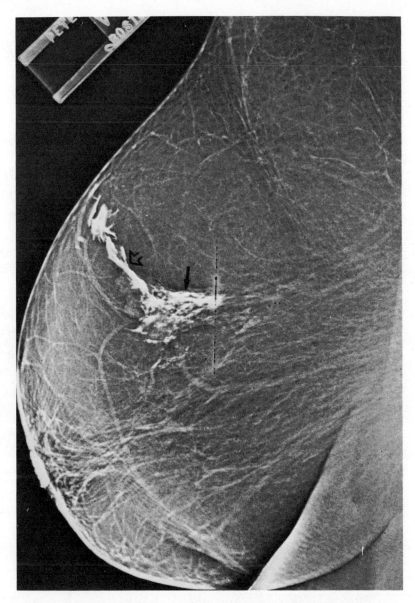

Figure 6–15. Methylene blue–contrast method of localization. Lateral xerogram with mixture of methylene blue and radiographic contrast material directly superimposed over area of suspicion (*solid arrow*). Linear track to skin surface (*open arrow*) allows for easier dissection to area.

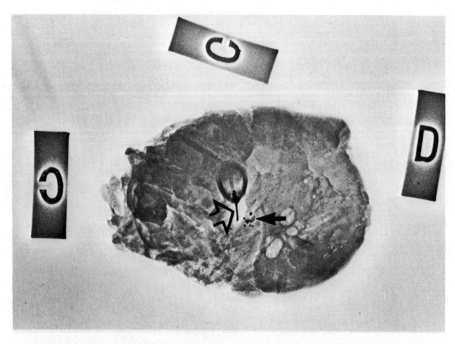

Figure 6–16. Specimen radiography. Specimen xerogram with 25-gauge needle (*open arrow*) marking area of suspicion (*closed arrow*) facilitates rapid frozen-section analysis.

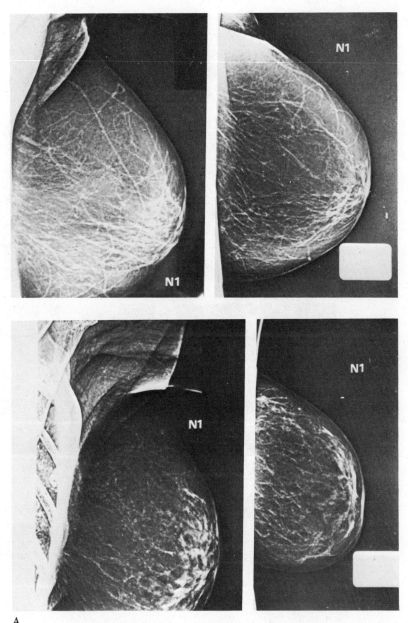

A
Figure 6–17. Risk patterns. A. N1. B. P1. C. P2. D. DY. (Courtesy of John Wolfe, M.D., Hutzel Hospital, Detroit, Mich.)

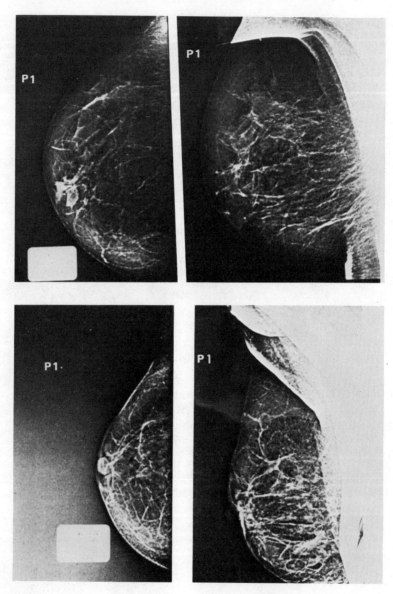

B

Figure 6–17 (Continued)

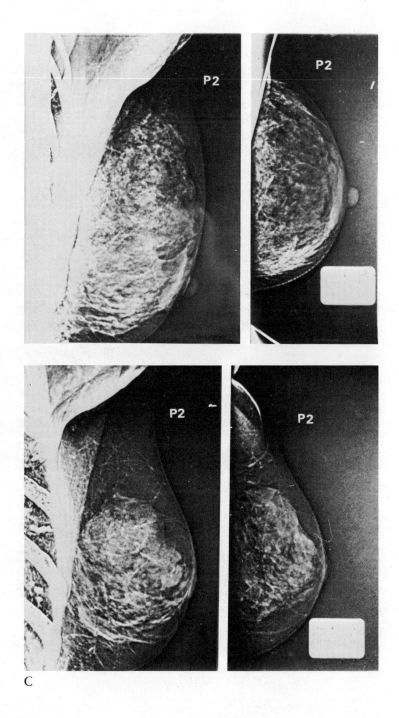

C

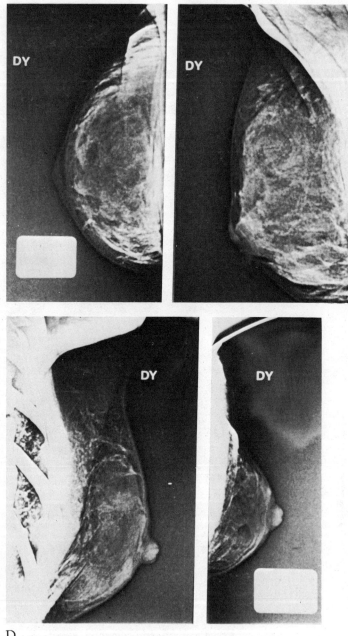

D

Figure 6–17 (Continued)

Differential Diagnosis

As explained previously, mammography is a potent means of detecting early malignant lesions. The decision tree that we and others involved with mammography follow entails a separation of the findings into three categories: benign, malignant, and questionable. In our reports, we always give a degree of certainty to lesions that are suspicious for malignancy. An irregularly shaped mass must always be biopsied. When we discover masses with smooth borders, mammograms cannot define with certainty their benignity, and their removal often becomes one of clinical judgment and conference between the surgeon and the radiologist. Those patients with less-clumped and/or symmetric calcifications may be followed at regular 6-month intervals. Close communication with the referring physician should be maintained for all patients being followed for questionable findings. Regardless of mammographic findings, any clinical change that raises the level of suspicion should lead to biopsy. The reverse is also true: Any suspicious mammographic findings should lead to biopsy even in the face of a completely negative physical exam.

One must keep in mind that mammography is not done to discourage biopsy, but quite the opposite. We can accept a slightly higher false positive rate for mammography as a screening examination in the hope of finding the very early nonclinical malignancy.

Practically speaking, several benign conditions may also closely mimic the findings of carcinoma, so that separation is not possible on radiographic grounds alone. Often, consultation with the clinician will make the correct diagnosis apparent in these patients. The remainder should undergo biopsy. A previous biopsy often creates a stellate mass as well as skin retraction and thickening. Because the findings may be identical to carcinoma, if the physician has not examined the patient or obtained a history of previous biopsy, he may identify the findings as carcinoma.

Trauma to the breast may produce either a hematoma or fat necrosis, either of which will appear as an irregular stellate mass. If a history of trauma is obtained, this can greatly aid in the differential diagnosis, although this history often cannot be elicited. If clinical findings are equivocal and trauma is the cause, the mammographic appearance may become less suspicious after 1 or 2 weeks; a repeat examination may be done after this time interval on selected patients. If no change is apparent, biopsy should be encouraged.

Although much less common, plasma cell mastitis and breast abscess may masquerade as inflammatory carcinoma and will produce a breast that is clinically inflamed and indurated. Plasma cell mastitis usually presents as an ill-defined asymmetric sub-areolar density with skin thickening; it often can only be separated from malignancy by biopsy. The history and clinical findings for abscess will usually lead the physician to prescribe a trial of antibiotics, which usually will produce complete remission of the abscess in 3 to 4 days.

Thermography

Thermography may best be defined as a method of mapping surface temperature variations that depends entirely upon radiated energy in the infrared spectrum. A detector within the apparatus converts the infrared radiation to an electrical output proportional to the emitted radiation. This information is then made available to some form of recording device. The degree of resolution (ability to identify small temperature differences) will change inversely with the speed at which the surface of interest is scanned; in other words, slower scanning produces greater resolution than more rapid scanning. The scan speed can range from a fraction of a second to minutes, with a compromise usually chosen. The sensitivity of the system relates to a differentiation between two temperature ranges approximately 0.1 to 0.5°C apart, over a range of 5 to 10°C. Black usually represents the cooler areas while white represents hot areas, with varying shades of gray in-between [22].

The room in which the examination is performed must be maintained at a fairly constant temperature, usually 20°C. The patient should be cooled with her arms on her head and allowed to reach the ambient temperature of the room before the procedure begins—5 to 10 minutes is adequate. Anterior and oblique images of each breast are obtained with the patient in an erect position with her arms still on her head.

The major feature to look for in a normal thermogram is

symmetry between the breasts. Several variations in normal vasculature may be encountered. These patterns correspond to subcutaneous veins, which are displayed as linear shadows over the breasts. Most commercial units will also provide a means for obtaining a direct temperature reading of an area of interest; again symmetry between the breasts should be present with regard to both vascular and nonvascular areas (Fig. 6–18). Its use as a diagnostic modality in breast cancer detection can be traced to Lawson and Gaston [37, 38], who demonstrated that breast cancers are warmer than adjacent tissue because of their increased blood supply and that the temperature of the skin in the area of palpable breast carcinomas is in general higher than the corresponding area of the contralateral breast. Subsequent studies confirmed this impression [18, 36, 42, 60].

Criteria for the abnormal breast thermogram have been reviewed and may be divided into vascular and nonvascular thermal patterns. The number of vessels should be relatively equal bilaterally. Vessels that are tortuous or serpiginous, or tend to cluster should be considered abnormal (Fig. 6–19). Nonvascular criteria include the "edge" sign, which is an asymmetric flattened breast contour or a localized protrusion within the breast. Any unilateral increase of 2 to 3°C between vessels is abnormal and is the major vascular thermal abnormality in thermograms. Nonvascular criteria include a diffuse surface temperature rise involving a part of or a whole breast, a localized increase of surface temperature, and a unilateral increase in areolar or subareolar temperature.

The procedure has the potential for great sensitivity in detecting abnormal heat patterns related to disease; however, it lacks specificity. Raskin and Martinez-Lopez [51], in a review of 1000 breast thermograms, found that almost 30 percent of benign breast conditions produced abnormal thermograms. An asymmetric venous pattern was associated with malignancy but was seen just as often in benign conditions. The diffuse increase in surface temperature involving more than a quadrant of the breast did correlate more frequently with large malignant lesions, however. These findings suggest that while the thermogram may be of value in patients with palpable lesions, it may not be specific enough for a screening examination in the asymptomatic person. Others [15, 49] have discovered similar findings when reviewing their material.

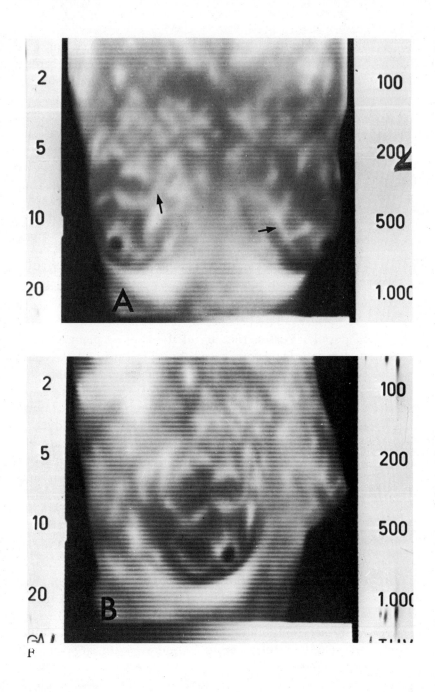

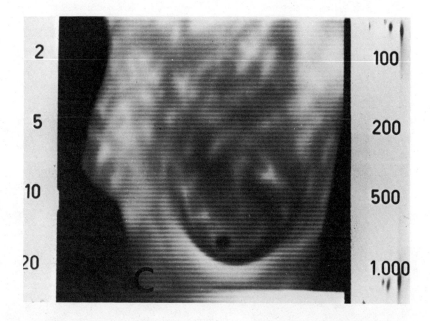

Figure 6–18. Normal thermogram. A. Anteroposterior view. Note similar vascular streaking (*arrows*) and symmetry. B. Right oblique view. C. Left oblique view. (Courtesy of Norman Sadowsky, M.D., Faulkner Hospital, Jamaica Plain, Mass.)

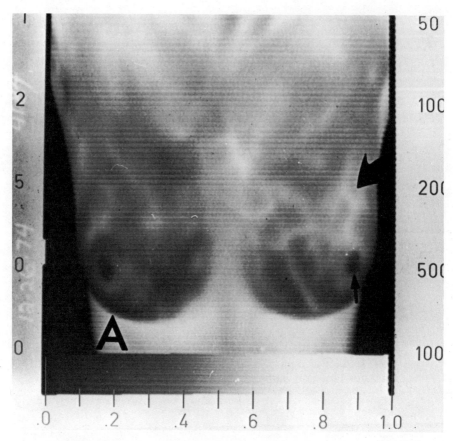

Figure 6–19. Thermogram showing carcinoma. (Courtesy of Norman Sadowsky, M.D., Faulkner Hospital, Jamaica Plain, Mass.) A. Thermogram in anteroposterior projection with asymmetric vascular pattern (*large curved arrow*). Note normal hypothermic area associated with nipple (*small arrow*). B. Right oblique view demonstrates left-sided increased heat and vascular pattern in comparison with the right side.

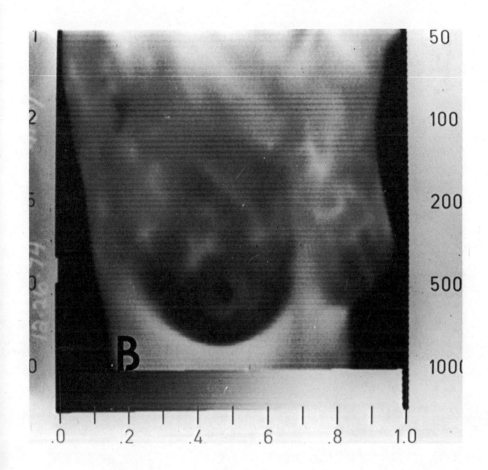

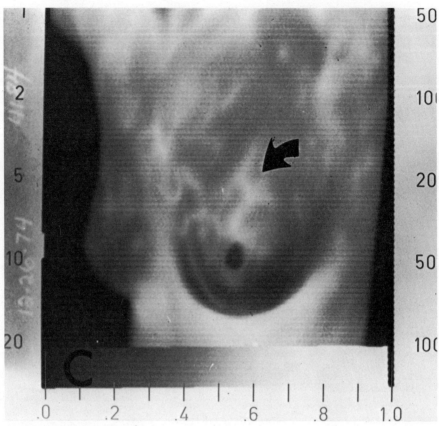

Figure 6–19 (Continued)

C. Left oblique view demonstrates left-sided increased heat and vascular pattern (*curved arrow*) in comparison with the right side. D. Lateral mammogram with clumped fine calcifications (*arrow*) in the same area of increased heat on the thermogram.

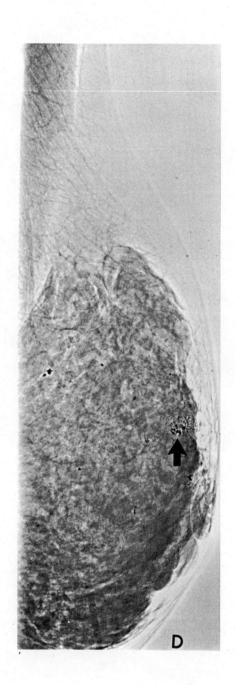

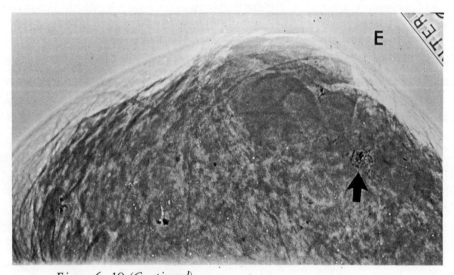

Figure 6–19 (Continued)
E. Craniocaudal mammogram with clumped fine calcifications
(*arrow*) in the same area of increased heat on the thermogram.

Since both the false positive and false negative rates are excessive, thermography's use as a screening tool does not appear to be appropriate. Its major thrust of application may be as a follow-up tool in treating the patient who already has had an initial physical examination, mammogram, and thermogram. The patient may then be followed at periodic intervals by means of physical examination and thermography. If any change shows up in either examination, mammography may then be obtained.

Ultrasound

Early in its development, diagnostic ultrasound was felt to be potentially useful for the diagnosis of breast disease. Indeed, Wild and his co-workers [64, 65], along with Howry and his group [25, 26], soon demonstrated the application of ultrasound in the differential diagnosis of breast lesions. The teams approached the problem of two-dimensional visualization in different ways: one with a water bath arrangement, the other with direct-contact scanning.

Since that time, many important contributions have been made to the understanding of the ultrasonic representation of breast tissue. In 1969, for example, Kelly-Fry and associates [30] were able to identify the various structural elements of the breast with ultrasound and to differentiate normal from abnormal tissue. In the early 1970s, Jellins and Kossoff and their group [29] in Australia reported on B-mode gray scale ultrasonic visualization of the breast, first with contact scanning [29] and then using an automated water bath scanner [35], thus ushering in the modern era of breast ultrasound.

As a noninvasive modality, ultrasound uses a short pulse of high-frequency sound (several million cycles per second) emitted into the body by a transducer. The higher this frequency, the greater the resolution of detail will be. However, higher frequencies also mean deeper penetration of the pulse into the body. A compromise is sought, therefore, between resolution and depth of penetration. The diagnostic range is usually from 2.25 MHz (2.25 million cycles/second) to 10 MHz, depending on the clinical situation.

As this pulse of sound travels through the tissues of the body, its speed is constant until it encounters tissue of different acoustic properties. At this interface of dissimilar acoustic impedance, a portion of the beam is reflected while the remainder continues through the material. The amplitude of the reflected echo is proportional to the difference of acoustic impedance or properties at the interface of the tissues. The greater this acoustic impedance difference, the greater the portion of the beam reflected and the lower the portion of the beam transmitted.

Another parameter of the ultrasound beam we must consider is that of attenuation. Basically, attenuation refers to the progressive weakening of the sound beam as it travels through tissue. The farther sound travels through tissue the weaker it gets. The attenuation of the ultrasonic beam depends on many factors, including type and density of the tissue and the number and type of echo interfaces in the tissue.

The criteria for detecting cystic and solid lesions can now be explained based on the facts briefly outlined above. Let us consider the path of an ultrasound beam through a cystic structure. The interfaces encountered by the beam are the near wall of the cyst, the fluid, and the far wall of the cyst. Thus, a portion of the beam is reflected at the near cyst wall, while the remainder passes into the cyst fluid. No echoes are reflected from the fluid because of its ultrasonically homogeneous nature. Thus the beam is transmitted with very little loss of strength (attenuation) to the far wall of the cyst with another echo reflected here, while the remainder is transmitted through the far wall of the cyst. The only two reflective surfaces encountered by the beam are the near and far walls of the cyst. Therefore, much of the original energy of the beam, because it is intact after passing through the cystic lesion, is still transmitted through the far wall so that echoes behind the cyst occur.

In contrast, a sound beam passing through a solid structure or mass produces findings opposite to those found with a cystic structure. Once again the first echo reflection would be from the near wall of the solid mass. However, the remaining transmitted beam would now encounter various interfaces in the solid structure not present in a cyst. As a result, multiple echoes would be reflected from the numerous different tissues with dissimilar acoustic properties, producing multiple echoes from within the mass. A corollary to this is the greater attenuation of the transmitted beam that occurs because of the energy absorption encountered when a sound beam passes through solid tissue. Because of this, echoes from the far side of a solid structure are markedly diminished or not present at all. The term *shadowing* is used when the echoes are not present at all.

With this basic understanding, then, we can summarize the ultrasonic characteristics of both cystic and solid masses (Figs. 6–20, 6–21). The cystic mass itself is echo-free, with production of strong echoes from the far side of the mass (the part farthest from the transducer); it is also sharply outlined. A solid mass has internal echoes, diminished echo production from the far side of the mass, and an indistinct outline.

Gradually, because of the mobility and pliability of the breast, contact B-scanning of the breast is being replaced by dedicated water path scanners using high-resolution transducers [45]. These scanners, which vary from manual to automated, have transducers capable of producing multiple images of the breast in several planes with intervals as close as 5 mm. With the newer versions, the patient is examined while she is in the prone position with her breasts suspended in water. It must be remembered that the ultrasound study produces a tomographic "slice" 1 to 3 mm in thickness. It is in this way that an ultrasound examination of the breast differs greatly from a radiographic examination, which represents superimposition of the entire breast contents in one image.

It is readily apparent that, as with x-ray mammography, there is no single, normal ultrasonic breast image because of the physiologic changes that occur with aging, childbirth, and lactation, as well as other factors. The skin is clearly outlined as a linear echogenic structure, immediately beneath which is the echo-poor layer of subcutaneous fat (Fig. 6–22). The parenchymal structure, composed of glandular tissue and fibrous tissue stroma interspersed with variable amounts of fat, is moderately echogenic, with a highly reflective retromammary fascia (Fig. 6–22). Generally, there is greater inhomogeneity of the parenchyma with aging, due to increased fat replacement. Echo-poor branching tubular structures extending from the nipple into the breast parenchyma probably represent periductal collagen or fat surrounding the ducts.

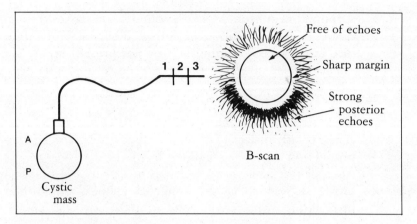

Figure 6–20. Ultrasonic features of a cystic lesion. The outlined lesion has few if any internal echoes. The outline of the lesion is sharply etched. There is strong echo production posterior to the lesion because of low sound absorption by the lesion.

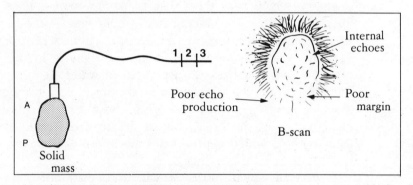

Figure 6–21. Ultrasonic features of a solid lesion. The lesion has multiple internal echoes. The margins are often poorly defined and irregular. There is an echo-poor area posterior to the mass because of high sound absorption by the lesion.

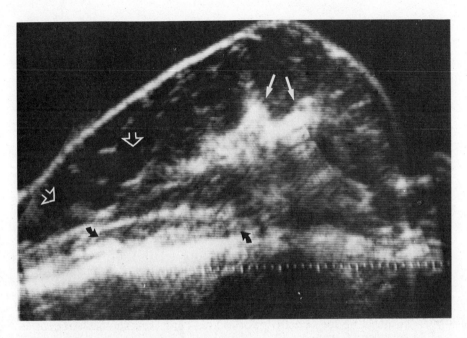

Figure 6–22. Normal breast architecture in a premenopausal patient. The echogenic glandular tissue (*straight arrows*) is roughly triangular in shape, relatively homogeneous, and radiating toward the nipple. Not infrequently, echo-free channels representing the ducts can be visualized. The echo-poor areas (*open arrows*) represent fat with interspersed fibrous tissue manifested by linear echogenic areas. The skin and retromammary fascia (*curved arrows*) are clearly delineated. (Courtesy of Barry Goldberg, M.D., Jefferson Memorial Hospital, Philadelphia, Pa.)

Fibrocystic disease of the breast encompasses a multitude of pathologic findings, and the ultrasonic patterns are therefore quite variable. In the dysplastic type, areas of very high echogenicity may coalesce to form bands that are interspersed with areas of fat of somewhat lower echogenicity. Varying numbers of echo-free cysts also may be present, occasionally with thickened, irregular walls that are probably secondary to chronic inflammation.

Kobayashi [32] developed ultrasonic diagnostic criteria for breast masses by reviewing the ultrasonic studies of 693 patients with palpable breast tumors that had been subsequently verified by excisional biopsy or mastectomy. He distinguished between the tumor characteristics in three major areas: the shape of the boundaries of the mass, the echo pattern within the mass, and the amplitude and configuration of the echoes posterior to the mass (Fig. 6–23).

In general, benign lesions are rounded, smooth, regular, and homogeneous or echo-poor, with strong enhancement of echoes posteriorly. In the case of a cyst, the echoes posterior to the mass most often have the shape of an inverted triangle due to differential reflection of the sound beam at the fluid–soft tissue interface. The typical cyst is solitary, variable in size, and echo-free, with well-defined margins and with lateral wall shadowing of the enhanced posterior echoes as described above (Fig. 6–24). In fibrocystic disease multiple cysts may be present, frequently with thickened, irregular walls. Benign solid masses differ from cysts in that they usually produce weak but uniform internal echoes with somewhat greater attenuation and less posterior enhancement (Fig. 6–25).

In contrast, the classic malignant lesion is irregular, infiltrating, and poorly circumscribed, with heterogeneous internal echoes and pronounced posterior shadowing due to strong attenuation (Fig. 6–26). Skin thickening [34] also may be detected ultrasonically, but it may be impossible to distinguish some malignant lesions, notably medullary carcinoma, from benign solid lesions. Fortunately cases of medullary carcinoma are infrequent, accounting for fewer than 10 percent of all malignant breast lesions. Other difficult diagnostic problems include abscesses, hematomas, scars, and fat necroses, all of which may be indistinguishable ultrasonically from malignant lesions. Furthermore, it

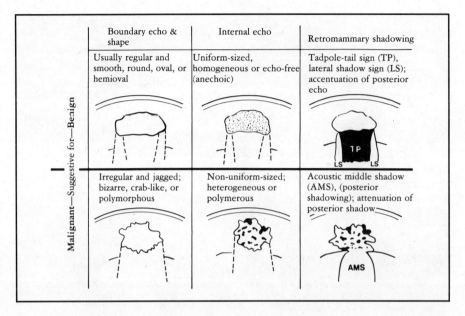

Figure 6–23. Schematic illustration of ultrasonic differential criteria. (Courtesy of Toshiji Kobayashi, M.D., University of Occupational and Environmental Health, Kitakyushu, Japan.)

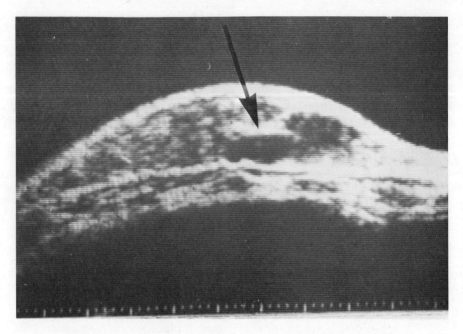

Figure 6–24. Benign cyst. The arrow points to an echo-free, somewhat flattened, sharply delineated area representing a breast cyst. Note the lack of shadowing behind the lesion. (Courtesy of Barry Goldberg, M.D., Jefferson Memorial Hospital, Philadelphia, Pa.)

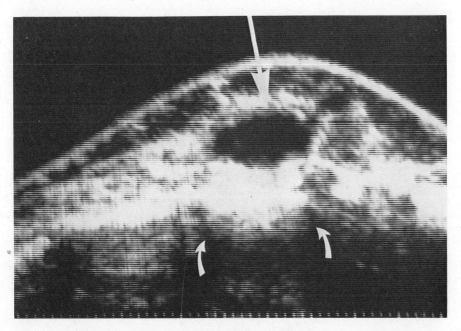

Figure 6–25. Fibroadenoma. Well-circumscribed solid lesion (*straight arrow*) at relatively medium-to-high gain setting with some shadowing posteriorly (*curved arrows*), as compared to the surrounding breast tissue. At still higher gain settings, the lesion would fill in with echoes. A fibroadenoma may be difficult or impossible to distinguish from a medullary carcinoma. (Courtesy of Barry Goldberg, M.D., Jefferson Memorial Hospital, Philadelphia, Pa.)

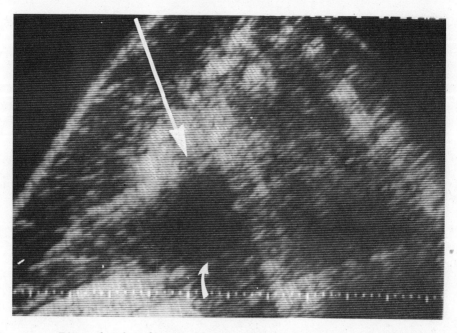

Figure 6–26. Infiltrating duct carcinoma. Poorly circumscribed, infiltrating echogenic structure (*straight arrow*) with lack of delineation of posterior wall with decreased sound penetration (*curved arrow*). These findings are typical for a malignant lesion, but, rarely, an inflammatory mass may produce a similar appearance. (Courtesy of Barry Goldberg, M.D., Jefferson Memorial Hospital, Philadelphia, Pa.)

is unlikely that microcalcifications can be detected with ultrasound unless they occur in large clusters that are echo-reflecting, producing posterior shadowing. Recently an attempt has been made to identify the ultrasonic equivalence of Wolfe's parenchymal patterns, but further studies are required [55].

Ultrasonic and radiographic examinations of the breast are just now beginning to be correlated. Jellins, Kossoff, and Reeve [28] recorded an accuracy of 98 percent for the detection of cysts when this was done. Kobayashi [31] reported on the combined results of several Japanese investigators; he found an average accuracy rate with ultrasound of 87 percent for malignant lesions and 80 percent for benign lesions in those patients referred because of palpable breast masses.

Harper and Kelly-Fry [21] reported quite favorably on their experience using a specially constructed automated breast scanner with over 400 patients referred for a variety of breast diseases. Some had ultrasound alone and others also had x-ray mammography. Cole-Beuglet and colleagues [9] compared ultrasound mammography with radiographic mammography in 705 of 1029 patients referred for examination; they reported the sensitivity for malignancy to be 69 percent for ultrasound mammography and 75 percent for x-ray mammography on independent readings. Most of the lesions detected by ultrasound, however, were palpable, with few lesions smaller than 2 cm in diameter.

In a similar study, Zusmer and co-workers [69] examined 293 referred patients independently with both ultrasound and xeroradiography. Twenty had radiographic evidence of malignancy; of those patients, 17 had ultrasonographic criteria for solid masses, 11 demonstrating signs of malignancy.

Certainly it appears that ultrasound of the breast holds great promise. It clearly has a role in distinguishing solid lesions from cysts and in the examination of radiographically dense breasts. In addition, ultrasound should be used as the first examination in women under the age of 30. However, further work must be carried out to improve the distinction between benign and malignant solid masses and ultimately to determine the exact role that ultrasound can play in the diagnostic workup of a patient with breast disease.

CT Scanning

Computerized axial tomography (CT) is an accepted and reliable technique for detecting intracranial pathology and is rapidly showing promise as a potent diagnostic tool in other areas of the body as well [1, 50]. Basically the scanner consists of a finely collimated x-ray beam opposite either a single detector moving in tandem with the source or multiple detectors arranged radially in a 360° circle. The latter method is the more modern and allows a scan to be completed in 2 to 4 seconds, obviating artifacts secondary to respiration. Thus, an 8-mm cross-sectional slice of the area of interest is obtained, which is the routine slice thickness employed. The area of consideration is broken up into a series of tissue cubes called pixels, each measuring $1.5 \times 1.5 \times$ the slice thickness. The number of these pixels is variable and depends on the area visualized. The x-ray absorption of structures within this pixel is critically analyzed to within a 1 to 2 percent accuracy. A cross-sectional image based on the various absorption coefficients is then reconstructed by means of the computer and displayed on a video screen for permanent recording either by disc or Polaroid print. The absorption coefficient for a particular area of interest can be plotted, and these numbers (at present termed *Hounsfield units*) correspond to the various densities observed in routine radiography. Originally the range was 1000 absorption units, from -500 represented by air to $+500$ represented by bone, with water density set at zero. Today the scale has been doubled so that -1000 represents air and $+1000$ represents bone. A further analysis of the technical aspects is beyond the scope of this chapter, but the basic concepts can be reviewed in Hounsfield's original description [24].

Initial studies using breast specimens from cadavers and surgical procedures revealed the accurate absorption data available but underlined the lack of anatomic resolution and overlap of malignant and benign processes with regard to absorption coefficients [12]. Absorption coefficients for malignant breast disease in vivo fell into a range of $+10$ to $+26.6$ units, using a -500 to $+500$ scale [2]. Although overlaps between certain types of fibrocystic disease and malignancy were appreciated, the use of contrast agents was beneficial in separating these areas of overlap [52]. Having a high absorption coefficient, the contrast agent will display areas of higher blood flow or regions extracting the contrast from the blood pool, or both. Due to the high degree of sensitivity of CT, small differences in contrast content are detectable.

With advances in CT technology, units have been constructed for breast use only. Scans are performed from the chest wall to the nipple. After both breasts have been examined, 300 cc of diatrizoate meglumine (Reno M Dip) are given by drip infusion within 10 minutes. The patient is then rescanned. In a recent study of 655 patients [8], the technique was felt to be superior to mammography, thermography, or physical examination for diagnosing both benign and malignant disease, especially in dense or fibrocystic breasts. All malignant lesions showed an increase in density of at least 5.2 percent measured in Hounsfield units. Enhancement was not as great for benign lesions.

This certainly is an area to be investigated intensively as a potential tool for more accurately defining malignant disease. The radiation dose per breast is approximately 240 mr, which may allow CT to be used as a screening technique.

References

1. Alfidi, R. J., Haaga, J., Meaney, T. F., et al. Computerized tomography of the thorax and abdomen: A preliminary report. *Radiology* 117:257, 1975.
2. Alfidi, R. J., MacIntyre, W. J., Meaney, T. F., et al. Experimental studies to determine application of CAT scanning to the human body. *A.J.R.* 124:199, 1975.
3. Bailar, J. C., III. Mammography: A contrary view. *Ann. Intern. Med.* 84:77, 1976.
4. Bailar, J. C., III. Screening for early breast cancer: Pros and cons. *Cancer* 39:2783, 1977.
5. Bailar, J. C., III. Mammographic screening: A reappraisal of benefits and risks. *Clin. Obstet. Gynecol.* 21:1, 1978.
6. Boice, J. D., Jr., and Manson, R. R. Breast cancer in women after repeated fluoroscopic examination of the chest. *J. Natl. Cancer Inst.* 59:823, 1977.
7. Breslow, L., Henderson, B., Massey, F., Jr., et al. Report of NCI ad hoc working group on the gross and net benefits of mammography in mass screening for detection of breast cancer. *J. Natl. Cancer Inst.* 59:475, 1977.
8. Chang, C. H. J., Sibala, J. L., Fritz, S. L., et al. Computed tomographic evaluation of the breast. *A.J.R.* 131:459, 1978.
9. Cole-Beuglet, C., Goldberg, B. B., Kurtz, A. B., et al. Ultrasound mammography: A comparison with radiographic mammography. *Radiology* 139:693, 1981.

10. Cooperman, A. M., Cook, S. A., Hermann, R. E., and Esselstyn, C. B., Jr. Preoperative localization of occult lesions of the breast. *Surg. Gynecol. Obstet.* 142:917, 1976.
11. Dodd, G. D., and Wallace, J. D. The venous diameter ratio in the radiographic diagnosis of breast cancer. *Radiology* 90:900, 1968.
12. D'Orsi, C. J., and Green, D. Computerized tomography and xeroradiography of breast specimens. *Breast* 2:27, 1976.
13. Egan, R. L. Experience with mammography in a tumor institution. *Radiology* 75:894, 1960.
14. Egan, R. L. Fundamentals of mammographic diagnoses of benign and malignant diseases. *Oncology* 23:126, 1969.
15. Feasey, C. M., Evans, A. L., and James, W. B. Thermography in breast carcinoma: Results of a blind reading trial. *Br. J. Radiol.* 48:791, 1975.
16. Frank, H. A., Hall, F. M., and Steer, M. L. Preoperative localization of nonpalpable breast lesions demonstrated by mammography. *N. Engl. J. Med.* 295:259, 1976.
17. Gallagher, H. S., and Martin, J. E. The study of mammary carcinoma by mammography and whole organ sectioning: Early observations. *Cancer* 23:855, 1969.
18. Gershon-Cohen, J., Berger, S. M., Haberman, J. A. D., and Barnes, R. B. Thermography of the breast. *A.J.R.* 91:919, 1964.
19. Hainline, S., Myers, L., McLelland, R., et al. Mammographic patterns and risk of breast cancer. *A.J.R.* 130:1157, 1978.
20. Hammerstein, G. R., Miller, D. W., White, D. R., et al. Absorbed radiation-dose in mammography. *Radiology* 130:485, 1979.
21. Harper, P., and Kelly-Fry, E. Ultrasound visualization of breast in symptomatic patients. *Radiology* 137:465, 1980.
22. Hodes, P. J., Wallace, J. D., and Dodd, G. D. Thermography. *Med. Clin. North Am.* 54:603, 1970.
23. Horns, J. W., and Arndt, R. D. Percutaneous spot localization of nonpalpable breast lesions. *A.J.R.* 127:253, 1976.
24. Hounsfield, G. N. Computerized transverse axial scanning (tomography): I. Description of system. *Br. J. Radiol.* 46:1016, 1973.
25. Howry, D. H., and Bliss, W. R. Ultrasonic visualization of soft tissue structures of the body. *J. Lab. Clin. Med.* 40:579, 1952.
26. Howry, D. H., Stott, D. A., and Bliss, W. R. The ultrasonic visualization of carcinoma of the breast and other soft tissue structures. *Cancer* 7:354, 1954.
27. Ingleby, A., and Gershon-Cohen, J. *Comparative Anatomy, Pathology, and Roentgenology of the Breast.* Philadelphia: University of Pennsylvania Press, 1960.
28. Jellins, J., Kossoff, G., and Reeve, T. S. Detection and classification of liquid-filled masses in the breast by gray scale echography. *Radiology* 125:205, 1977.
29. Jellins, J., Kossoff, G., Reeve, T. S., et al. Ultrasonic grey scale visualization of breast disease. *Ultrasound Med. Biol.* 1:393, 1975.

30. Kelly-Fry, E., Gibbons, L. V., and Kossoff, G. Characterization of breast tissue by ultrasonic visualization methods (abstract). Proceedings of the 78th meeting of the Acoustical Society of America, San Diego, Calif., 1969. P. 30.
31. Kobayashi, T. Ultrasonic diagnosis of breast cancer. *Ultrasound Med. Biol.* 1:383, 1975.
32. Kobayashi, T. Gray-scale echography for breast cancer. *Radiology* 122:207, 1977.
33. Koehl, R. H., Snyder, R. E., Hutter, R. V. P., and Foote, F. W., Jr. The incidence and significance of calcifications within the operative breast specimens. *Am. J. Clin. Pathol.* 53:3, 1970.
34. Kopans, D. B., Meyer, J. E., and Proppe, K. H. The double line of skin thickening on sonograms of the breast. *Radiology* 141:485, 1981.
35. Kossoff, G., Carpenter, D. A., Robinson, D. E., et al. A new multitransducer water coupling echoscope (abstract no. 17). Proceedings of the Second European Congress of Ultrasonics in Medicine, Munich, Germany, May 1975.
36. Lapayowker, M. S., Barash, I., Byrne, R., et al. Criteria for obtaining and interpreting breast thermograms. *Cancer* 38:1931, 1976.
37. Lawson, R. Implications of surface temperatures in the diagnosis of breast cancer. *Can. Med. Assoc. J.* 75:309, 1956.
38. Lawson, R. N., and Gaston, J. P. Temperature measurements of localized pathological processes. *Ann. N.Y. Acad. Sci.* 121:90, 1964.
39. Leborgne, R. Diagnostico des los tumores de la mama por la radiografia simple. *Arch. Urug. Med.* 37:44, 1950.
40. Leborgne, R. L. Diagnosis of tumors of the breast by simple roentgenography. *A.J.R.* 65:1, 1951.
41. Libshitz, H. I., Feig, S. A., and Fetouh, S. Needle localization of nonpalpable breast lesions. *Radiology* 121:557, 1976.
42. Lloyd-Williams, K., Lloyd-Williams, F. J., and Handley, R. S. Infra-red thermometry in the diagnosis of breast disease. *Lancet* 2:1378, 1961.
43. MacDonald, I. The Breast. In J. Davis (Ed.), *Christopher's Textbook of Surgery* (9th ed.). Philadelphia: Saunders, 1968.
44. Mandell, L., Rosenbloom, M., and Naimark, A. Are breast patterns a risk index for breast cancer? A reappraisal. *A.J.R.* 128:547, 1977.
45. Maturo, V. G., Zusmer, N. R., Gilson, A. J., et al. Ultrasound of the whole breast utilizing a dedicated automated breast scanner. *Radiology* 137:457, 1980.
46. McGregor, D. H., Land, C. E., Choi, K., et al. Breast cancer incidence among atomic bomb survivors, Hiroshima and Nagasaki, 1950–69. *J. Natl. Cancer Inst.* 59:799, 1977.
47. Millis, R. R., Davis, R., and Stacey, A. J. The detection and significance of calcifications in the breast: A radiological and pathological study. *Br. J. Radiol.* 49:12, 1976.

48. Moskowitz, M., Gartside, P., Gardella, L., et al. The breast cancer screening controversy: A perspective. *A.J.R.* 129:537, 1977.
49. Moskowitz, M., Milbrath, J., Gartside, P., et al. Lack of efficacy of thermography as a screening tool for minimal and stage I breast cancer. *N. Engl. J. Med.* 295:249, 1975.
50. New, P. F. J., Scott, W. R., Schnur, J. A., et al. Computerized axial tomography with the EMI scanner. *Radiology* 110:109, 1974.
51. Raskin, M. M., and Martinez-Lopez, M. Thermographic patterns of the breast: A critical analysis of interpretation. *Radiology* 121:553, 1976.
52. Reese, D. F., Carney, J. A., Grisvold, J. J., et al. Computerized reconstructive tomography applied to breast pathology. *A.J.R.* 126:406, 1976.
53. Rogers, J. V., Jr., and Powell, R. W. Mammographic indications for biopsy of clinically normal breasts: Correlation with pathologic findings in 72 cases. *A.J.R.* 115:794, 1972.
54. Rosen, P. P., Snyder, R. E., and Robbins, G. Specimen radiography for nonpalpable breast lesions found by mammography: Procedures and results. *Cancer* 34:2028, 1974.
55. Rubin, C. S., Kurtz, A. B., Goldberg, B. B., et al. Ultrasonic mammographic parenchymal patterns: A preliminary report. *Radiology* 130:515, 1979.
56. Salomon, A. Beitragezur pathologie und klinik des mammakarzinoms. *Arch. Klin. Chir.* 1:573, 1913.
57. Shapiro, S., Strax, P., and Venct, L. *Periodic Breast Cancer Screening in Presymptomatic Detection and Early Diagnosis.* London: Sir Isaac Pitman and Sons, 1968. P. 203.
58. Shapiro, S., Strax, P., and Venct, L. Periodic breast cancer screening in reducing mortality from breast cancer. *J.A.M.A.* 215:1777, 1971.
59. Shore, R. E., Hempelmann, L. H., Kowaluk, E., et al. Breast neoplasms in women treated with x-rays for acute postpartum mastitis. *J. Natl. Cancer Inst.* 59:813, 1977.
60. Swearingen, A. G. Thermography: Report of the radiographic and thermographic examination of the breast of 100 patients. *Radiology* 85:818, 1965.
61. Update on mammography. *ACR Bull.* 32:1, 1976.
62. Wanebo, C. K., Johnson, K. G., Sato, K., and Thorslund, T. W. Breast cancer after exposure to the atomic bombings of Hiroshima and Nagasaki. *N. Engl. J. Med.* 279:667, 1968.
63. Warren, S. L. A roentgenologic study of the breast. *A.J.R.* 24:113, 1930.
64. Wild, J. J., and Neal, D. The use of high frequency ultrasonic waves for detecting changes of texture in living tissues. *Lancet* 1:655, 1951.
65. Wild, J. J., and Reid, J. M. Echographic visualization of lesions of the living intact human breast. *Cancer Res.* 14:277, 1954.
66. Wolfe, J. N. Xeroradiography of the breast. *Oncology* 23:113, 1969.

67. Wolfe, J. N. Breast patterns as an index of risk for developing breast cancer. *A.J.R.* 126:1130, 1976.
68. Wolfe, J. N., Dooley, R. P., and Harkins, L. E. Xeroradiography of the breast: A comparative study with conventional film mammography. *Cancer* 28:1569, 1971.
69. Zusmer, N. R., Goddard, J., Maturo, V. G., et al. Automated sonomammographic-xeromammographic-pathologic correlations in the assessment of carcinoma of the breast. *J. Ultrasound Med.* 1:19, 1982.

William D. Kaplan

7. Radionuclide Diagnosis and Management of Carcinoma of the Breast

Although virtually any organ system within the body can be imaged with radionuclides, the diagnostic tracer studies in patients with carcinoma of the breast have centered about scintigraphy of the bones and liver. Indeed, these two imaging tests can represent up to three quarters of the studies performed in an oncology setting. Because these tests are at the same time noninvasive and sensitive for detecting tumor sites, bone and liver-spleen scans have been fully integrated into the clinical evaluation of patients either suspected or known to be harboring breast cancer. In this chapter I will summarize the key methods for best employing these tests and for interpreting the data from these studies. Finally, some of the newer radionuclide examinations now available will be reviewed.

Radionuclide Identification of Primary Breast Malignancy

Although the major application of radionuclide studies has been the definition of metastatic disease, a sizable experience has focused on attempts to define the primary lesion in patients with carcinoma of the breast. A number of tracers have been evaluated as potential tumor-specific radionuclides. Initial approaches involved the intravenous administration of radiophosphorus or radiocesium followed by external counting with a scintillation probe placed over the breast suspected of harboring malignant tissue [53, 60]. Early experiences with external imaging, using a rectilinear scanner, attempted to define sites of selective uptake within breast tumors after the intravenous administration of radioactive potassium, mercury, bismuth, rubidium, or iodine [6, 29, 39, 73, 74].

The widespread use of technetium-99m (^{99m}Tc) as pertechnetate in the evaluation of brain malignancies led to the chance observation of its sequestration within breast tissue. Although early reports indicated a moderate sensitivity for detecting tumor

Table 7-1   Results of [67]Ga Imaging in 125 Patients with Primary and Metastatic Breast Cancer [64]

Time of Evaluation	Organ	% True Positive Scans
Preoperative	Breast	52
Postoperative	Bone	65
	Lung	35
	Brain	20
	Liver	8

[15, 63, 77], a false positive rate that approached 30 percent suggested that there were clinical limitations to the use of this tracer as an aid in the differential diagnosis of breast masses [63].

With the use of ^{99m}Tc-labeled bone agents, a plethora of reports appearing in the literature also suggested that this radiopharmaceutical could be used in the detection of breast malignancies [8, 21, 69, 72, 78]. Unfortunately, not only was the bone agent noted to sequester within tumor (whether primary or metastatic to the breast) [71] but also within 45 percent of benign breast masses [21] and in nonmalignant, non-breast-related changes within the thorax [38].

The use of gallium-67 (^{67}Ga) citrate as a general tumor scanning agent has been proposed in a number of clinical reviews [33, 42, 49]. However, the role of this radiotracer for differentiating both primary and metastatic deposits from breast carcinoma has been less enthusiastically received [63]. In a prospective series in which 125 patients were referred for preoperative and postoperative evaluation of breast cancers, the diminished sensitivity for detecting both the primary and secondary foci by gallium scanning suggested limited utility for this agent (Table 7-1) [64].

A more promising application of gallium scintigraphy in the evaluation of patients with breast cancer may lie in the definition of tumor involvement within the mediastinum [64]. In a review of 29 patients, 88 percent of the women with biopsy-proven mediastinal involvement showed positive gallium uptake in this anatomic site. Only one patient showed a false positive scan; that is, abnormal uptake in an area proven by biopsy to be normal. Of importance, in 43 percent of the "gallium-positive" patients the chest x-rays were completely normal. In a group of patients with no postoperative evidence of mediastinal disease, 95 percent had normal gallium scans. In the one patient who had positive mediastinal uptake with the radionuclide, the scan returned to normal following a course of chemotherapy. This information suggests that when radiographs are suspicious for mediastinal involvement, and mediastinoscopy for biopsy has not been or cannot be performed, ^{67}Ga citrate imaging may be particularly useful in delineating the presence of mediastinal tumor.

Attempts at using radiolabeled tumor-seeking antibodies to define sites of primary neoplasia have received recent attention, although experiences with carcinoma of the breast have been limited [32]. Whether the use of monoclonal antibodies [7] will prove fruitful or whether metastatic foci with their high levels of tumor-associated antigen will be better defined by radiolabeled antibody imaging [22] remains to be seen.

Of the many radionuclides used over the past years in attempts to preoperatively localize sites of primary breast malignancy, none has been shown to be clinically efficacious. It appears that, for the time being anyway, tracer techniques have neither the sensitivity nor the specificity to be practical for screening or for differentiating between malignant and benign breast masses.

Assessing the Extent of Disease Preoperatively
Bone
Radionuclide imaging of the skeletal system by defining blood flow, osteoblastic activity, and bone turnover [17] can allow identification of skeletal metastases months to years before changes can be seen radiographically; loss of calcium content of bone must approach 50 percent before one can expect to see x-ray change [27]. Significantly less in the way of mineral loss and subsequent bony repair will initiate an abnormal focus on bone scan. Indeed, although the scan and x-rays most frequently agree (both being either positive or negative in 80 percent of cases), in approximately 15 percent of cases only the radionuclide bone scan will define a skeletal abnormality.

The bone agents in general use today employ ^{99m}Tc to label phosphorus-containing ligands. The theoretical mechanism of action centers about the adsorption of the phosphate moiety to crystallites of bone [41]. Approximately half of the injected radiopharmaceutical rapidly associates with the bony matrix within the first hour after administration; that tracer remaining in the circulation must be eliminated by the kidneys over the next few hours before a bone-to-background ratio of sufficient magnitude is achieved. This high ratio of skeletal-to-background activity is needed in order to define regions of increased bone turnover that may represent metastases. Patients are routinely asked to drink liquids during the 2- to 4-hour interval between injection and imaging; this promotes renal clearance of circulating, non-skeletal-bound radionuclide.

The radionuclide definition of skeletal lesions is closely related to the type of instrumentation used [66]. The traditional rectilinear scanner employs a small moving crystal for defining emitted gamma rays as the detector head moves line-by-line over the length of the patient. The newer Anger-type cameras make use of a wide, 15-inch crystal such that large areas of the skeletal system—for example, the entire thorax or pelvis—can be imaged on a single view within minutes. Although cameras are also capable of producing a "total body" image similar to that achieved with the rectilinear scanner, there are clinically significant differences between the images created on the two instruments; these are related to the number of counts per square centimeter of film. Rectilinear bone images, for example, can represent only about 30 to 50 percent of the count density obtained when using Anger cameras. This difference in count densities can be responsible theoretically for an increased incidence of false negative studies when rectilinear scanners are the only instrument employed for bone scanning (Fig. 7-1).

A similar potential for false negative studies relates to the use of "limited" bone scans. In many institutions the bone scan includes only the axial skeleton. Reports defining the distribution of metastatic foci [70, 76] indicate that the extremities are involved by metastases with a frequency approaching 25 percent (Fig. 7-2). In the management of patients with breast carcinoma metastatic to bone, the pretreatment baseline scan should define *all* lesions, so that on follow-up studies one is able to differentiate between new and old sites of skeletal metastases.

Although the bone scan is extremely sensitive for detection

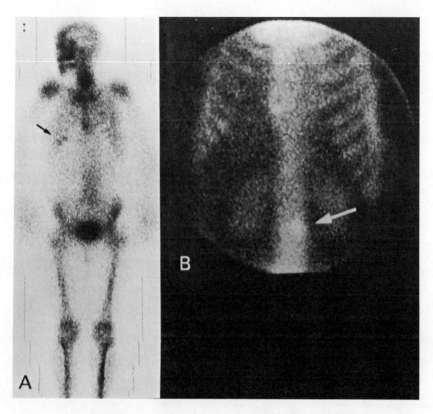

Figure 7–1. Anterior total body rectilinear scan (A) shows subtle rib uptake (*arrow*). Anger camera scintiphoto (B) obtained to better define ribs shows additional lesion in lumbar spine.

Anterior

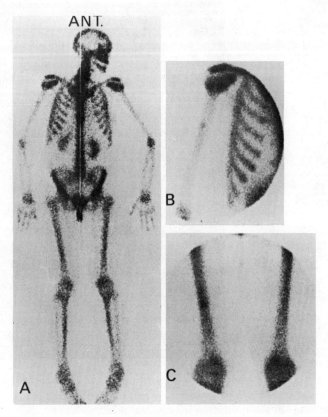

Figure 7-2. A total body Anger camera bone scan (A) reveals a suspicious abnormal focus in the right midhumerus and right midfemur. High resolution views (B, C) confirm these foci, which proved to be metastases from breast carcinoma.

of disease, a lack of specificity implies that a positive scan does not necessarily reflect a site of skeletal tumor. Indeed, many pathologic but nonmalignant entities are capable of manifesting foci of increased uptake (Table 7-2) [61]. This only emphasizes the necessity of interpreting the positive bone scan along with an x-ray; it is suggested that all scintigraphic abnormalities be at least correlated with the concomitant radiograph during the initial patient visit.

The presence of a normal scan should not preclude obtaining selected radiographs. Purely lytic and slow-growing lesions may escape radionuclide detection. Pain, if apparent, may indicate specific sites for x-ray evaluation [54]. Particular attention must be directed to weight-bearing areas and the cervical spine, anatomic locations at which a pathologic fracture carries significant clinical implications (Figs. 7-3, 7-4). Even in asymptomatic patients with negative scans, baseline chest, skull, pelvic, and thoracic-spine x-rays are reasonable studies to have for future comparison.

Whether or not the referring physician should expect a positive bone scan is closely related to the clinical stage of the breast malignancy at the time the patient is first seen. Initial reports of bone scan imaging in patients with breast cancer implied that even in the early stages of the disease, positive skeletal involvement could be expected in up to 30 percent of cases [19, 35, 65]; indeed, more recent series confirm that philosophy [48]. Results of other studies, however, including the experiences at our institution, indicate that the yield of a positive bone scan in patients with Stage I or II carcinoma of the breast will be quite low, on the order of less than 5 percent [31, 50, 56].

Table 7-2 Some Non-malignant Causes of Increased Uptake on Bone Scans [61]

Osseous	Soft Tissue
Fracture	Calcified tendinitis
Arthritis	Healing and postoperative scars
Osteomyelitis	Injection sites
Osteoporosis	Myositis ossificans
Paget's disease	Myocardial infarcts
Renal osteodystrophy	Postradiation therapy

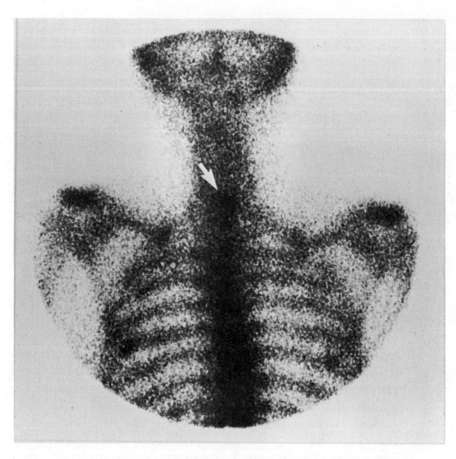

Figure 7–3. Posterior view of the cervical and upper thoracic spine on bone scan. The degree of radionuclide uptake at C-7 (*arrow*) is normal to minimally increased.

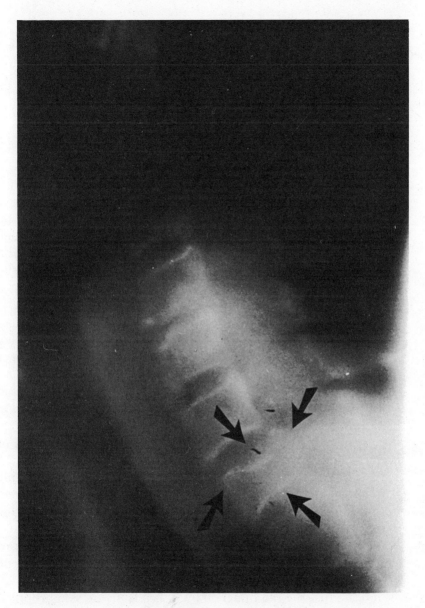

Figure 7–4. A lateral cervical spine film reveals a compression fracture of C-7 with depression of the upper and lower articular margins (*arrows*). This finding is compatible with a pathologic fracture.

This is not to imply that there is no utility in obtaining bone scans in patients with early stage disease at the time they are first seen. It is frequently invaluable for the nuclear radiologist to have at hand high-quality pretreatment scintiscans for comparison when patients return for follow-up views with a question of new skeletal metastases or for assessment of the effects of chemotherapy.

In summary, ^{99m}Tc-phosphate total body Anger camera bone images provide a reliable and sensitive indicator of bone turnover. It must be stressed that all radionuclide abnormalities must be correlated with radiographs and that in spite of a negative bone scan, areas that are clinically symptomatic should be radiographed to rule out potential sites of lytic disease. Although early stages of breast cancer are infrequently associated with skeletal abnormalities, a baseline study can frequently have significant bearing on future therapeutic manipulations.

Liver

Although the liver does not represent the most common site of metastatic involvement from carcinoma of the breast, it is involved frequently enough to deserve special attention [1]. An abnormal physical examination coupled with elevated values in liver function tests usually directs the physician toward suspicion of hepatic metastases. However, the presence of tumor in livers of normal size [62] and in patients who evidence normal or only minimal nonspecific abnormalities in their liver function tests [40] indicates that additional modalities for monitoring potential hepatic metastases should be considered. For this reason, the clinician has relied heavily upon noninvasive imaging techniques to detect these foci of hepatic neoplasia.

Results of a comparative study, in which the sensitivity of computed tomography, ultrasound, and radionuclide imaging of the liver for defining intrahepatic metastases was evaluated, indicate that the radionuclide liver scan is the most appropriate *initial* imaging procedure for detecting liver tumor [2, 13] (Table 7-3). In part, its appropriateness is because the radionuclide liver scan is able to portray the entire liver, from the subphrenic space to the inferior edge of the right and left hepatic lobes. It can be completed within approximately 45 minutes from the time of injection. The information obtained is not dependent upon slice thickness, as it is with computed tomography, nor

Table 7-3   Sensitivity and Specificity for the Image Detection of
Pathologically Proven Intrahepatic Metastases [2]

Modality	Sensitivity	Specificity
Computed axial tomography	0.82	0.69
Ultrasound	0.50	0.75
Radionuclide imaging	0.82	0.83

are regions of the liver obscured by overlying gas or bony structures, as occurs with ultrasound [36]. In addition, the radionuclide evaluation of the liver is not operator-dependent, inasmuch as image collection is fully automated.

The radionuclide liver scan is a sensitive test for detecting hepatic abnormalities; this has been especially true since the advent of newer instrumentation and concomitant higher resolution Anger cameras (Figs. 7-5, 7-6). Particularly apparent when using the Anger camera is the elegant appreciation of superficial lesions and surface anatomy. This feature can be important in identifying metastatic deposits that are implanted upon the serosa of the liver.

The classic description of metastatic lesions involving the liver is that of an intrahepatic focal defect. Following intravenous administration of ^{99m}Tc-labeled sulfur colloid, approximately 85 percent of the tracer is normally sequestered within functioning reticuloendothelial (RE) cells of the liver. When hepatic parenchyma is replaced by tumor, this is manifested on scintiscan as a focal absence of RE uptake (Fig. 7-6).

A word of caution, however, in using scintigraphic information that indicates an abnormal liver in patients with carcinoma of the breast: A recent study indicates that patterns compatible with diffuse parenchymal disease (such as hepatomegaly, heterogeneous distribution of intrahepatic tracer, and shifts of radiocolloid to the extrahepatic RE system) may potentially represent hepatic involvement by metastatic carcinoma from the breast (Fig. 7-7). This scan pattern of diffuse disease of the liver can be associated with a metastatic etiology in approximately half of all cases [24]. Therefore, with underlying breast malignancy, both carcinomatosis [11] and cirrhosis should be considered when the nuclear medicine report indicates diffuse hepatic involvement.

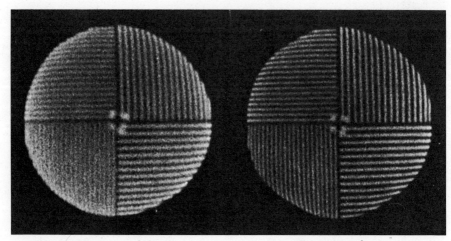

Preupgrade   Postupgrade

Figure 7–5. Scintiphotos of a lead bar phantom obtained preupgrade and postupgrade of an Anger camera. The finest bar spacing of 3 mm (*left lower quadrant*) is quite clearly seen following instrument upgrade (postupgrade).

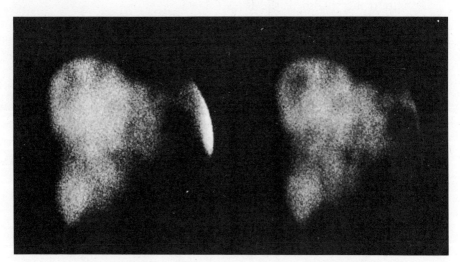

Preupgrade   Postupgrade

Figure 7–6. Anterior 630,000 count views of a patient liver preupgrade and postupgrade. Patient was imaged in the late morning and then 2 hours later (without reinjection of radiocolloid) after the old camera components were replaced. Note the better definition of pathologic foci in image on the right.

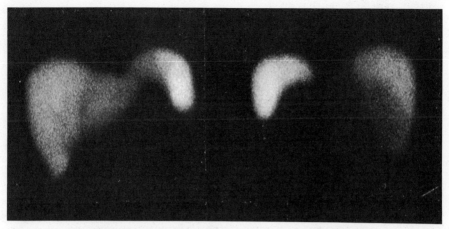

Anterior   Posterior

Figure 7–7. Anterior and posterior views of the liver in a patient
with carcinoma of the breast. Note the absence of intrahepatic focal
defects; however, there is heterogeneous distribution of
radiocolloid in the liver with a shift to the spleen. Biopsy revealed
extensive metastases.

In patients in whom the radionuclide liver scan demonstrates heterogeneity, there appears to be little value in utilizing ultrasound in an attempt to define the existence of focal intrahepatic abnormalities [16]. To illustrate this, at our institution when 31 patients with radionuclide changes compatible with diffuse disease were evaluated, only one patient demonstrated a focal lesion at the time of ultrasound examination. In this patient the tumor focus was localized to the most lateral aspect of the left hepatic lobe and could only be appreciated on radionuclide study during a retrospective analysis.

To date, no extensive information exists regarding the propensity for hepatic involvement in relation to the clinical stage of breast cancer. Since a trend similar to that manifested in patients with skeletal metastases is found when correlating clinical stage of disease with liver scans, it is suggested that a baseline radionuclide liver-spleen study be obtained at the time the patient is initially seen. This scintigraphic information will be invaluable for future comparative studies.

Assessing the Extent of Disease Postoperatively
Bone
The need for baseline pretreatment skeletal images of high quality must again be stressed. Without benefit of a previous study, a subtle abnormality seen on a follow-up bone scan could be misconstrued to represent a new metastatic lesion. When an available baseline examination is checked, the abnormality can frequently be seen on pretreatment images. In such cases, the radiographs become critically important in guiding the clinician toward appropriate therapy.

The question of frequency with which follow-up bone scans should be obtained has been addressed in a number of studies [14, 20, 31, 47, 56]. It appears that approximately 25 percent of patients with Stage I and II disease show tumor recurrence in bone within the first 18 months after they were first seen. Those with Stage III and IV disease tend to show a 75 percent or greater recurrence rate within a similar time period. These findings suggest that total body bone scans obtained every 6 months during the first 2 years followed by annual images over the next 3 years are the most appropriate scanning regimen for identifying skeletal recurrence.

On occasion more frequent imaging intervals may produce striking and unsuspected findings. Figure 7-8 shows the baseline and follow-up images performed over a 3-week interval. The repeat study obtained for the purpose of defining a biopsy site for data on estrogen receptivity shows the appearance of a new rib lesion in a patient with untreated carcinoma of the breast. Radiographs taken at the time of both radionuclide studies were normal.

Of interpretive importance is the recognition of the potential for a flare phenomenon that has been associated with therapy [5, 59]. In general, sequential scintiscans in patients undergoing chemotherapy tend to show a relative decrease in the degree of focal uptake as the most common manifestation of healing (Fig. 7-9). A transient increase in the relative intensity of bone lesions may be a normal phenomenon, however, reflecting the increased blood flow and osteoblastic activity of healing (Fig. 7-10), and this should not necessarily be misconstrued as progressive skeletal disease. This manifestation of healing has been associated with the use of both hormonal therapy and chemotherapy.

It should be noted that the relative intensity of a lesion on bone scan refers to the ratio of intensities of abnormal bone to adjacent normal bone; it is this ratio of abnormal-to-normal bone that is compared to subsequent ratios in differentiating between healing and tumor-involved bone. The comparison of how "hot" a lesion is on one day as compared to how hot it is 1 month later is an unreliable indicator of either healing or tumor growth, since the intensity settings selected for the camera frequently vary on a daily basis.

Only with close follow-up of a large series of patients will the common patterns of the bone scan response to therapy be accurately defined. Until this time, sequential bone images that show increased uptake following therapeutic manipulation should be interpreted with caution and in conjunction with appropriate clinical information.

The relationship between skeletal pain and scintigraphic findings has been discussed in a number of series [9, 10, 18]. Between 15 and 40 percent of asymptomatic patients have been

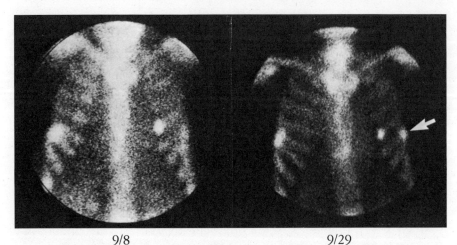

9/8   9/29

Figure 7–8. Sequential anterior thorax images obtained 3 weeks apart show the rapid appearance of a metastatic lesion in the rib (*arrow*).

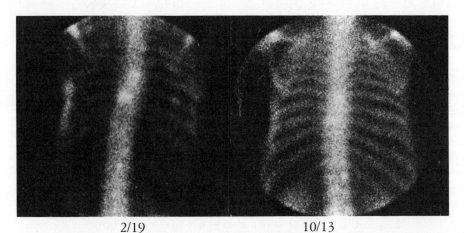

2/19   10/13

Figure 7–9. Posterior views of the midthoracic spine on bone scans obtained approximately 8 months apart. Note the decrease in focal uptake in the lateral ribs and vertebral bodies on the 10/13 study following chemotherapy for carcinoma of the breast.

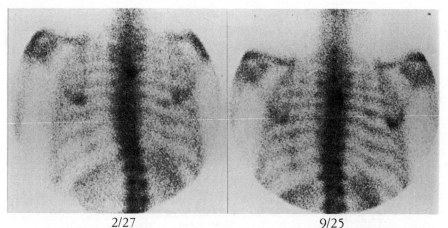

2/27   9/25

Figure 7–10. Posterior images of the thoracic spine taken 7 months apart. Note the increased uptake in the upper thoracic vertebral body on the follow-up image. Radiographs showed sclerosis, which is compatible with a positive chemotherapeutic effect.

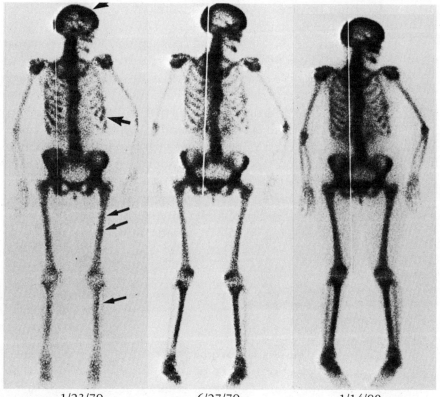

1/23/79   6/27/79   1/14/80

Figure 7–11. Sequential total body Anger camera bone scans obtained over a 1-year interval. Note on the study of 1/23/79 the abnormal skull, ribs, and left lower extremity lesions (*arrows*). These abnormalities resolved with chemotherapy, resulting in a normal bone scan on 1/14/80. At no time did any of the radiographs of these areas show abnormalities.

found to have positive bone scans. A review of the experiences at the Peter Bent Brigham Hospital [55] indicates that although 48 percent of patients manifested pain in an area shown to be abnormal on bone scan, 44 percent had no evidence of pain in abnormal regions. The other 8 percent of patients had pain located in areas remote to those defined as abnormal on the radionuclide study. Of patients with normal bone scans, 91 percent had no clinical evidence of pain. Consequently it would appear that the presence or absence of bone pain is an unreliable indicator in the evaluation of skeletal metastases. I would like to again stress the necessity of obtaining radiographs of symptomatic areas of the skeletal system even in patients with normal bone scans. Purely lytic or slow-growing metastatic foci, or both, can escape scintigraphic definition, and only by x-ray examination can treatment failures and sites of potential pathologic fractures be adequately identified.

Although the most reassuring scintigraphic and radiographic patterns of a positive chemotherapeutic effect are those showing diminished relative uptake of radionuclide within focal skeletal sites and x-rays that show progression from purely lytic lesions to those that are sclerotic, it appears that this latter radiographic finding may be manifested infrequently [19]. Indeed, cases have been seen of clinical improvement manifested only by laboratory tests and scintiscans with no evidence of x-ray change during the entire course of therapy (Fig. 7-11). Although initial sequential radionuclide skeletal imaging may show persistent abnormal foci with normal x-rays, in time, repeat bone scans in the responding patient will frequently show diminished focal tracer uptake. It is this spectrum of scan findings that, when correlated with serial blood chemistries and tumor markers, will strongly support the clinical impression of tumor regression rather than progression.

Liver
As mentioned earlier, the overall sensitivity of radionuclide liver imaging for detection of intrahepatic abnormalities is high; when correlated with clinicopathologic findings, detection approaches 92 percent [25]. In addition, when the results of liver function tests and serum levels of tumor-associated antigen are combined with the imaging result, the sensitivity for detecting intrahepatic metastases is even greater [51, 75]. These findings suggest that

the radionuclide liver scan can be used with confidence for the early detection of new metastatic liver disease and for following the effects of therapeutic manipulations in sites of known liver metastases.

When parallel hole collimation is utilized during Anger camera imaging of the liver, an accurate portrayal of intrahepatic focal abnormalities can be obtained, and the sequential sizing of these lesions as a function of therapy can be monitored [80] (Fig. 7-12). It must be cautioned that not uncommonly both tumor markers *and* liver scintiscans may be necessary to best define the true clinical response. Recent information correlating intrahepatic tumor with variations in carcinoembryonic antigen (CEA) levels indicates that the latter may less accurately reflect actual tumor response [12].

However, the absence of change in an intrahepatic focal abnormality has been noted occasionally during sequential scintigraphy in patients who clearly showed both a clinical response and a response in tumor markers as monitored by measurements of circulating CEA levels (Fig. 7-13). For this reason, nonalteration of an intrahepatic focal lesion's size should not immediately be thought to represent a treatment failure. On the other hand, an increase in size of an intrahepatic focal lesion and the appearance of new focal abnormalities within the liver are most consistent with progressive tumor involvement.

A potential cause of a false positive liver scan is the effect of chemotherapeutic agents upon the intrahepatic distribution of ^{99m}Tc-sulfur colloid. Short-term cancer chemotherapy has been shown to produce alterations in the radiocolloid distribution in up to one half of patients examined [45]. That the changes seen on scintiscan were mainly those compatible with a diffuse pattern of liver involvement is particularly significant in view of the frequency with which breast carcinoma can produce just such a scintigraphic picture.

Solitary focal abnormalities within the liver occur infrequently, with the incidence reported to be approximately 2 to 3 percent [23, 62]. If, on review, the baseline liver-spleen scan has been normal, then a new solitary focal defect is a grave finding. However, if no earlier study is available, or should the baseline radionuclide evaluation similarly identify a single focal abnormality, a careful evaluation must be performed to exclude a benign etiology.

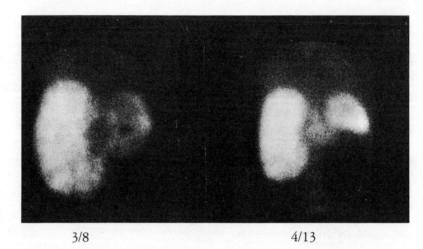

3/8   4/13

Figure 7–12. Two anterior images of the liver in a patient with carcinoma of the breast. By using parallel hole collimation the marked resolution of intrahepatic tumor over the 5-week interval can be accurately sized for comparative purposes.

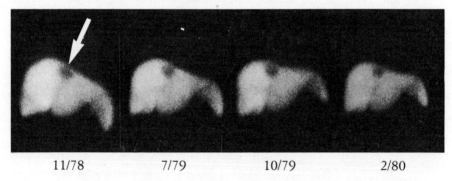

11/78   7/79   10/79   2/80

Figure 7–13. Sequential anterior scintiphotos of the liver in a patient with carcinoma of the breast metastatic to liver. The solitary focal abnormality (*arrow*) has shown no significant change in size or configuration over 15 months of follow-up. The patient is currently without evidence of active disease after chemotherapy.

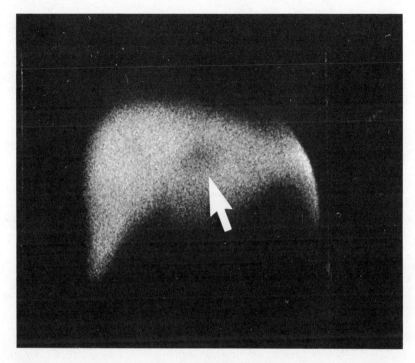

Figure 7–14. On this anterior view of the liver, we see a single focal intrahepatic defect in the left lobe (*arrow*).

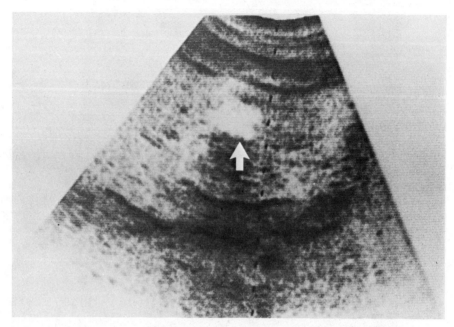

Figure 7–15. Ultrasound examination of the defect seen in Figure 7–14 defines its etiology as a prominent hepatic vein (*arrow*).

In a general hospital setting, approximately one half of these solitary focal abnormalities have had a benign cause [23]. In our experience within an oncology hospital, approximately 40 percent of single focal hepatic abnormalities have been associated with a benign etiology. If one considers only those focal lesions that are completely surrounded by normal-appearing liver parenchyma and are geographically removed from normal anatomic regions of diminished uptake (i.e., gallbladder fossa and porta hepatis), approximately 15 percent of these focal changes will be shown to be due to nonmalignant causes. Therefore, a simple additional diagnostic study such as an ultrasound evaluation of the area in question can lead to a final diagnosis of a benign lesion in a patient highly suspect for new intrahepatic metastatic focus (Figs. 7-14, 7-15).

To summarize, both skeletal and hepatic radionuclide evaluations have been shown to be extremely sensitive indicators of the presence of pathology; however, neither test has a degree of specificity sufficient to allow absolute statements to be made regarding the presence of tumor. Data from both examinations need to be closely correlated with additional diagnostic modalities, that is, radiographs, liver chemistries, and, when indicated, ultrasound examination and computed tomography. In addition, it must be appreciated that metastatic involvement of the bone and liver can be a long-term and slow-growing process. The changes manifested on scintiscan of either positive chemotherapeutic response or tumor growth can be expected to be quite variable. Use of sequential imaging to monitor the spectrum of disease will allow the clinician to best characterize the course of the tumor growth in each patient. Meticulous attention to each individual scintigraphic abnormality as defined on sequential images will be invaluable in allowing the physician to make the best clinical decision.

New Applications
Planning Radiation Therapy Portals
The technique of radionuclide lymphoscintigraphy has allowed the clinician to define the position and functional integrity of a previously anatomically silent lymphatic system [28]. By subcostal injections of small amounts of ^{99m}Tc-labeled radiocolloid, the normal anatomic pathways of lymphatic drainage through

the internal mammary lymph node chain can easily be defined (Fig. 7-16). Based upon this technique, a method for the three-dimensional localization of the internal mammary nodes has been made available for purposes of planning radiation therapy portals [26]. The clinical importance of this technique centers about previous conceptions of the normal position of the internal mammary lymph nodes. In a study by Rose and co-workers [67], the authors indicated that up to 40 percent of radiation therapy treatment plans would have been inadequate, under-dosing one or more lymph nodes, had not the precise anatomic location of these structures been defined prior to treatment.

In a review of the results of internal mammary lymph node imaging in 400 patients at our institution, we assessed the three-dimensional position of over 2600 lymph nodes. It was found that approximately 20 percent of the internal mammary nodes located within the second through the fourth interspaces were positioned *at or beyond* the expected 3-cm depth and distance off the midline [43]. These numbers correspond almost exactly to those previously cited [67] in a smaller series of patients.

This tracer technique also holds promise for defining potential spread or recurrence of tumor within the internal mammary chain in patients with carcinoma of the breast. Neoplastic involvement of the lymphatics has been associated with diminished intranodal concentration of radiocolloid and has impeded progression of the tracer through the lymph channel (Fig. 7-17). The ultimate role of this technique in defining recurrent disease awaits additional data related to sensitivity and specificity.

Dynamic Radionuclide Studies

With the use of an Anger camera, numerous dynamic radionuclide studies can easily be performed. In general, all of these examinations entail the intravenous (IV) injection of the diagnostic radionuclide followed by rapid image collection (1-2 frames/sec). Diagnostic results are generally available in a matter of minutes. Images depicting blood flow through the venous and arterial tree can be noninvasively collected and displayed. This technique lends itself to the evaluation of entities such as superior vena caval (SVC) obstruction.

Although the relative incidence of SVC obstruction due to

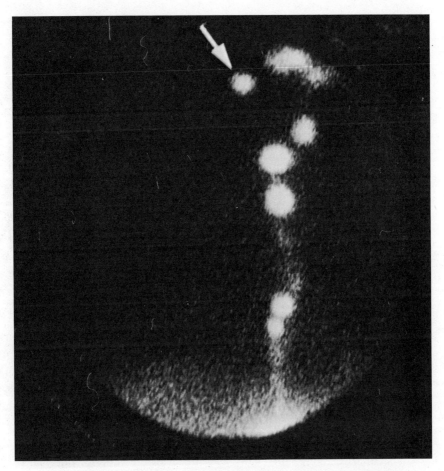

Figure 7–16. An anterior view of the thorax showing uptake of radiocolloid in the internal mammary lymph nodes. The liver is seen at the inferior aspect of the image; the sternal notch is identified by a radioactive marker (*arrow*).

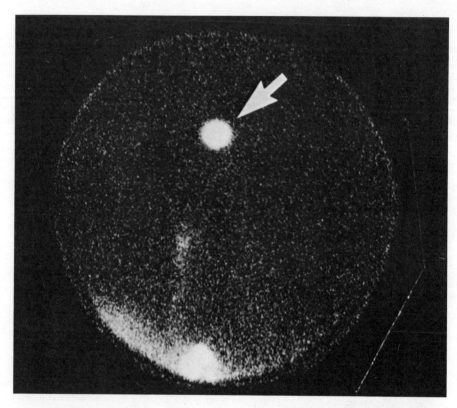

Figure 7–17. An anterior view of the thorax in a patient with carcinoma of the breast involving the internal mammary lymph nodes. Note the absence of focal nodal accumulation, poor filling of the lower lymphatic chain, and cut-off of the superior one half of the channel. The sternal notch is identified by a radioactive marker (*arrow*). Activity in the lower aspect of the image represents the injection site.

metastatic disease from all causes approximates only 7 percent [52], the clinical ramifications are significant. Injections of the large volumes of iodinated contrast material needed for x-ray evaluation of acute obstruction can cause significant side effects. The radionuclide vena caval study is an elegant method for assessment. The IV injection of only small volumes of tracer can accurately depict the pathways of venous return to the right heart, allowing visualization of collateral flow in pathologic states [58, 68] (Fig. 7-18).

With the rapid improvement in instrumentation and advances in radiopharmaceuticals, cardiovascular nuclear medicine has recently undergone dramatic growth. Radiotracer techniques for estimation of myocardial blood flow, metabolism, and cardiac hemodynamics are now accepted in routine clinical practice. With these techniques we are able to provide sensitive tools to aid in the assessment of both normal and abnormal cardiac function [37].

The use of doxorubicin hydrochloride (Adriamycin) in patients with carcinoma of the breast has been shown to be highly efficacious [34]. However, use as long-term therapy may be limited by the development of cardiomyopathies [57]. By employing quantitative radionuclide angiocardiographic techniques, changes in ejection fraction can be identified in patients at risk for drug-induced cardiotoxicity. These radionuclide-identified changes can be defined prior to clinical manifestations and overt congestive failure [4]. Although the initial techniques for radionuclide assessment of cardiac function were based on "first pass" studies of tracer transiting the left ventricle, current techniques employ electrocardiographically gated equilibrium techniques for ventriculography. With this approach, serial studies in multiple projections are obtained, and parameters such as regional ejection fraction (of either the right or left ventricle), regional wall motion abnormalities, and variations in cardiac function both at rest and exercise allow accurate, noninvasive assessment of cardiac function.

Although traditionally the noninvasive nature of radionuclide flow studies has relied upon intravenous administration of tracers, with the advent of intraarterial hepatic artery catheters for chemotherapy of carcinoma of the breast metastatic to the liver, radionuclide evaluation of arterial blood flow has now become a practical test [44]. By means of intraarterial infusion of ^{99m}Tc-

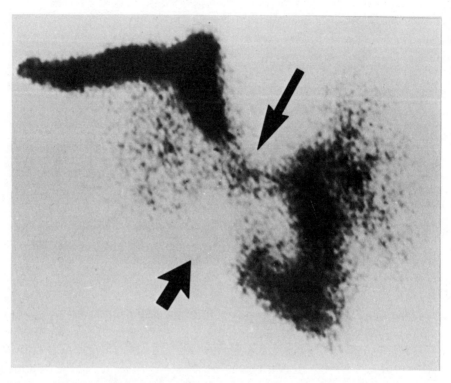

Figure 7–18. An anterior view of the thorax during a first pass of radionuclide through the right heart. The superior vena cava shows obstruction (*upper arrow*). Tracer flow into the right heart, pulmonary artery, and lungs shows decreased pulmonary perfusion of the right lung (*lower arrow*) due to mediastinal and perihilar tumor.

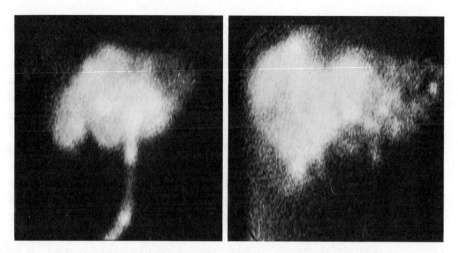

Figure 7–19. Anterior images of the intrahepatic distribution of radioaggregates administered via femoral to hepatic artery at a flow rate of 21 ml per hour. The two studies were obtained 4 days apart with no intervention between examinations. Note marked alteration in the pattern of flow. Lack of tumor response in patients such as these may well be due to ineffective drug delivery even with the catheter in an optimal position.

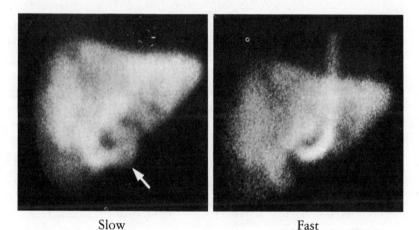

Slow   Fast

Figure 7–20. Slow intraarterial infusion of 21 ml per hour (*left*) does not allow adequate perfusion and drug delivery to tumor focus (*arrow*); adequate perfusion is seen only with fast (1.0 ml/sec) infusion.

macroaggregated albumin via an automated pump mechanism, radiotracer distribution within the liver at flow rates of 10 to 21 ml/per hour (the identical rates used to administer chemotherapy) has allowed predictive statements regarding potential response to treatment to be made [46] (Fig. 7-19). Additional information relevant to patient management centers around identifying those individuals at risk for systemic toxicity due to extrahepatic drug flow and arteriovenous shunting as manifested by pulmonary uptake of radioaggregates, and around the assessment of optimal flow rate of drug administration based on perfusion patterns of radioaggregates administered at a variety of infusion speeds (Fig. 7-20).

Throughout this chapter a number of features have emerged that characterize the application of radionuclide evaluation to patients with carcinoma of the breast. These studies, while noninvasive and sensitive, lack specificity. This latter point suggests the need for the clinician to interact with the nuclear medicine department to best integrate the implication of all test results. It is only through an understanding of whether or not the radionuclide report represents a patient assessment based on a combination of radiographic, ultrasonic, and computed tomographic information that the referring physician can best direct his continuing efforts in either the preoperative or postoperative care of his patient.

Although we have stressed the use of imaging of bone and liver, the two organ systems most commonly involved by metastatic breast cancer, there exists a host of other tracer studies with an equally high degree of sensitivity for evaluating the presence of metastases. These would include use of the radionuclide brain scan and the new hepatobiliary agents for use in patients with elevated serum bilirubins that may preclude routine x-ray examinations. The reader may wish to consult numerous review articles [3, 30, 79] to put these diagnostic studies in perspective.

A final point should be made concerning the written requisition for radionuclide studies. The nuclear medicine physician is able to answer only those questions that are asked. When the referring physician supplies a clinical history and a clinical question on the requisition, the scan report will best represent data at will be most useful in the total management of the patient with carcinoma of the breast.

Acknowledgments

The author wishes to thank Elaine N. Dufresne and Christopher Black for their technical assistance, John Buckley and Deborah Hansen for their photography and artwork, and Barbara Connolly for her assistance in the preparation of the manuscript.

References

1. Abrams, H. L., Spiro, R., and Goldstein, N. Metastases in carcinoma: Analysis of 1,000 autopsied cases. *Cancer* 3:74, 1950.
2. Alderson, P.O., Adams, D.F., McNeil, B.J., et al. Comparison of CT, ultrasound, and radionuclide scanning in the assessment of hepatic metastases. In preparation.
3. Alderson, P. O., Gado, M. H., and Siegel, B. A. Computerized cranial tomography and radionuclide imaging in the detection of intracranial mass lesions. *Sem. Nucl. Med.* 7:161, 1977.
4. Alexander, J., Dainiak, N., Berger, H. J., et al. Serial assessment of doxorubicin cardiotoxicity with quantitative radionuclide angiocardiography. *N. Engl. J. Med.* 300:278, 1979.
5. Alexander, J. L., Gillespie, P. J., and Edelstyn, G. A. Serial bone scanning using technetium-99m-diphosphonate in patients undergoing cyclical combination chemotherapy for advanced breast cancer. *Clin. Nucl. Med.* 1:13, 1976.
6. Baker, W. H., Nathanson, I. T., and Selverstone, B. Use of radioactive potassium (K-42) in the study of benign and malignant breast tumors. *N. Engl. J. Med.* 252:612, 1955.
7. Ballou, B., Levine G., Hakala, T. R., et al. Tumor localization detected with radioactively labeled monoclonal antibody and external scintigraphy. *Science* 206:844, 1979.
8. Berg, G. R., Kalisher, L., Osmond, J. D., et al. ^{99m}Tc-diphosphonate concentration in primary breast carcinoma. *Radiology* 109:393, 1973.
9. Blair, J. S. G. Does early detection of bone metastases by scanning improve prognosis in breast cancer? *Clin. Oncol.* 1:185, 1975.
10. Bonadonna, G., Brusamolino, E., Valagussa, P., et al. Combination chemotherapy as an adjuvant treatment in operable breast cancer. *N. Engl. J. Med.* 294:405, 1976.
11. Borja, E. R., Hori, J. M., and Pugh, R. P. Metastatic carcinomatosis of the liver mimicking cirrhosis: Case report and review of the literature. *Cancer* 35:445, 1975.
12. Bronstein, B. R., Steele, G. D. Jr., Ensminger, W., et al. The use and limitations of serial plasma carcinoembryonic antigen (CEA) levels as a monitor of changing metastatic liver tumor volume in patients receiving chemotherapy. *Cancer* 46:266, 1980.
13. Bryan, P. J., Dinn, W. M., Grossman, Z. D., et al. Correlation of computed tomography, Gray scale ultrasonography, and radionuclide imaging of the liver in detecting space-occupying processes. *Radiology* 124:387, 1977.

14. Burkett, F. E., Scanlon, E. F., Garces, R. M., et al. The value of bone scans in the management of breast cancer patients. *Surg. Gynecol. Obstet.* 149:523, 1979.
15. Cancroft, E. T., and Goldsmith, S. J. ^{99m}Tc-pertechnetate scintigraphy as an aid in the diagnosis of breast masses. *Radiology* 106:441, 1973.
16. Chafetz, N., Taylor, A., Alazraki, N. P., et al. The heterogeneous liver scan: Ultrasound correlation. *Radiology* 130:201, 1979.
17. Charkes, N. D. Mechanisms of skeletal tracer uptake. *J. Nucl. Med.* 20:794, 1979.
18. Charkes, N. D., Malmud, L. S., Caswell, T., et al. Preoperative bone scans; use in women with early breast cancer. *J.A.M.A.* 233:516, 1975.
19. Citrin, D. L., Bessent, R. G., Greig, W. R., et al. The application of the ^{99m}Tc-phosphate bone scan to the study of breast cancer. *Br. J. Surg.* 62:201, 1975.
20. Citrin, D. L., Tormey, D. C., and Carbone, P. P. Implications of the ^{99m}Tc-diphosphonate bone scan on treatment of primary breast cancer. *Cancer Treat. Rep.* 61:1249, 1977.
21. Clyne, C. A. C., Perry, P. M., Gibson, A., et al. ^{99m}Tc-polyphosphate uptake by breast tumors. *Br. J. Surg.* 65:773, 1978.
22. DeLand, F. H., Kim, E. E., Corgan, R. L., et al. Axillary lymphoscintigraphy by radioimmunodetection of carcinoembryonic antigen in breast cancer. *J. Nucl. Med.* 20:1243, 1979.
23. Drum, D. E. Optimizing the clinical value of hepatic scintiphotography. *Sem. Nucl. Med.* 8:346, 1978.
24. Drum, D. E., and Beard, J. M. Scintigraphic criteria for hepatic metastases from cancer of the colon and breast. *J. Nucl. Med.* 17:677, 1976.
25. Drum, D. E., and Christacopoulos, J. S. Hepatic scintigraphy in clinical decision making. *J. Nucl. Med.* 13:908, 1972.
26. Dufresne, E. N., Kaplan, W. D., Zimmerman, R. E., et al. The application of internal mammary lymphoscintigraphy to radiation therapy planning. *J. Nucl. Med.* 21:697, 1980.
27. Edelstyn, G. A., Gillespie, P. J., and Grebbel, F. S. The radiologic demonstration of osseous metastases: Experimental observations. *Clin. Radiol.* 18:158, 1967.
28. Ege, G. N. Internal mammary lymphoscintigraphy. The rationale, technique, interpretation, and clinical application: A review based on 848 cases. *Radiology* 118:101, 1976.
29. Eskin, B. A., Parker, J. A., Bassett, J. G., et al. Human breast uptake of radioactive iodine. *Obstet. Gynecol.* 44:398, 1974.
30. Fordham, E. W. The complementary role of computerized axial transmission tomography and radionuclide imaging of the brain. *Sem. Nucl. Med.* 7:137, 1977.
31. Gerber, F. H., Goodreau, J. J., Kirchner, P. T., et al. Efficacy of preoperative and postoperative bone scanning in the management of breast carcinoma. *N. Engl. J. Med.* 297:300, 1977.

32. Goldenberg, D. M., DeLand, F., Kim, E., et al. Use of radiolabeled antibodies to carcinoembryonic antigen for the detection and localization of diverse cancers by external photoscanning. *N. Engl. J. Med.* 298:1384, 1978.

33. Hayes, R. L. The medical use of gallium radionuclides: A brief history with some comments. *Sem. Nucl. Med.* 8:183, 1978.

34. Henderson, I. C., and Canellos, G. P. Cancer of the breast. The past decade. *N. Engl. J. Med.* 302:17, 78, 1980.

35. Hoffman, H. C., and Marty, R. Bone scanning: Its value in the preoperative evaluation of patients with suspicious breast masses. *Am. J. Surg.* 124:194, 1972.

36. Holm, H. H., Rasmussen, S. N., and Kristensen, J. K. Errors and pitfalls in ultrasonic scanning of the abdomen. *Br. J. Radiol.* 45:835, 1972.

37. Holman, B. L. Cardiac imaging in nuclear medicine. *Radiology* 133:709, 1979.

38. Isitman, A. T., Komaki, S., and Holmes, R. A. A benign uptake of ^{99m}Tc-polyphosphate after radical mastectomy. *Radiology* 110:159, 1974.

39. Jacobstein, J. G., and Quinn, J. L. Uptake of ^{206}Bi-citrate in carcinoma of the breast. *Radiology* 107:677, 1973.

40. Jhingran, S. G., Jordan, L., Johns, M. F., et al. Liver scintigrams compared with alkaline phosphatase and BSP determinations in the detection of metastatic carcinoma. *J. Nucl. Med.* 12:227, 1971.

41. Jones, A. G., Francis, M. D., and Davis, M. A. Bone scanning: Radionuclide reaction mechanisms. *Sem. Nucl. Med.* 6:3, 1976.

42. Kaplan, W. D., and Adelstein, S. J. The radionuclide identification of tumors. *Cancer* 37:487, 1976.

43. Kaplan, W. D., Connolly, B. T., and Rose, C. M. Internal mammary lymphoscintigraphy: The radionuclide localization of lymph nodes in 400 patients. In preparation.

44. Kaplan, W. D., D'Orsi, C. J., Ensminger, W. D., et al. Intraarterial radionuclide infusion: A new technique to assess chemotherapy perfusion patterns. *Cancer Treat. Rep.* 62:699, 1978.

45. Kaplan, W. D., Drum, D. E., Lokich, J. J. The effect of cancer chemotherapeutic agents on the liver-spleen scan. *J. Nucl. Med.* 21:84, 1980.

46. Kaplan, W. D., Ensminger, W. D., Smith, E. H., et al. Radionuclide angiography to predict patient response to hepatic artery chemotherapy. *Cancer Treat. Rep.* 64:1217, 1980.

47. Khandekar, J. D. Role of routine bone scans in operable breast cancer: An opposing viewpoint. *Cancer Treat. Rep.* 63:1241, 1979.

48. Komake, R., Donegan, W., Manoli, R., et al. Prognostic value of pretreatment bone scans in breast carcinoma. *A.J.R.* 132:877, 1979.

49. Larson, S. M. Mechanism of localization of gallium-67 in tumors. *Sem. Nucl. Med.* 8:193, 1978.

50. Lentle, B. C., Burns, P. E., Dierich, H., et al. Bone scintiscanning

in the initial assessment of carcinoma of the breast. *Surg. Gynecol. Obstet.* 141:43, 1975.

51. Liewendahl, K., and Schauman, K. O. Statistical evaluation of liver scanning in combination with liver function tests. *Acta Med. Scand.* 192:395, 1972.

52. Lokich, J. J., and Goodman, R. Superior vena caval syndrome: Clinical management. *J.A.M.A.* 231:58, 1975.

53. Low-Beer, B. V. A., Bell, H. G., McCorkle, H. J., et al. Measurement of radioactive phosphorus in breast tumors in situ; a possible diagnostic procedure. *Radiology* 47:492, 1946.

54. McNeil, B. J. Rationale for the use of bone scans in selected metastatic and primary bone tumors. *Sem. Nucl. Med.* 8:336, 1978.

55. McNeil, B. J. Personal communication, 1980.

56. McNeil, B. J., Pace, P. D., Gray, E. B., et al. Preoperative and follow-up bone scans in patients with primary carcinoma of the breast. *Surg. Gynecol. Obstet.* 147:745, 1978.

57. Minow, R. A., Benjamin, R. S., and Lee, E. T. Adriamycin cardiomyopathy—risk factors. *Cancer* 39:1397, 1977.

58. Miyamae, T. Interpretation of ^{99m}Tc superior vena cavograms and results of studies in 92 patients. *Radiology* 108:339, 1973.

59. Nesto, R. W., Cady, B., Oberfield, R. A., et al. Rebound response after estrogen therapy for metastatic breast cancer. *Cancer* 38:1834, 1976.

60. Nishiyama, H., Moskowitz, M., Saeujer, E. L., et al. Lack of specificity for detection of breast lesions with radioactive cesium chloride. *Surg. Gynecol. Obstet.* 143:229, 1976.

61. O'Mara, R. E. Bone scanning in osseous metastatic disease. *J.A.M.A.* 229:1915, 1974.

62. Ozarda, A., and Pickren, J. The topographic distribution of liver metastases: Its relation to surgical and isotopic diagnosis. *J. Nucl. Med.* 3:149, 1962.

63. Richman, S. D., Brodey, P. A., Frankel, R. S., et al. Breast scintigraphy with ^{99m}Tc-pertechnetate and ^{67}Ga-citrate. *J. Nucl. Med.* 16:293, 1975.

64. Richman, S. D., Ingle, J. N., Levenson, S. M., et al. Usefulness of gallium scintigraphy in primary and metastatic breast carcinoma. *J. Nucl. Med.* 16:996, 1975.

65. Roberts, J. G., Gravelle, I. H., Baum, M., et al. Evaluation of radiography and isotopic scintigraphy for detecting skeletal metastases in breast cancer. *Lancet* 1:237, 1976.

66. Rollo, D. F., and Hoffer, P. Comparison of whole-body-imaging methods. *Sem. Nucl. Med.* 7:315, 1977.

67. Rose, C. M., Kaplan, W. D., Marck, A., et al. Parasternal lymphoscintigraphy: Implications for the treatment planning of internal mammary lymph nodes in breast cancer. *Int. J. Radiat. Oncol. Biol. Phys.* 5:1849, 1979.

68. Rosenthall, L. Radionuclide venography using technetium-99m-pertechnetate and the gamma ray scintillation camera. *A.J.R.* 97:874, 1966.

69. Serafini, A. N., Raskin, M. M., Zand, L. C., et al. Radionuclide breast scanning in carcinoma of the breast. *J. Nucl. Med.* 15:1149, 1974.

70. Shirazi, P. H., Rayudu, G. V. S., and Fordham, E. W. [18]F bone scanning: Review of indications and results of 1,500 scans. *Radiology* 112:361, 1974.

71. Shultz, M. M., Morales, J. O., Fishbein, P. G., et al. Bilateral breast uptake of ^{99m}Tc-polyphosphate in a patient with metastatic adenocarcinoma. *Radiology* 118:377, 1976.

72. Siegel, M. E., Friedman, B. H., and Wagner, H. N., Jr. A new approach to breast cancer; breast uptake of ^{99m}Tc-HEDSPA. *J.A.M.A.* 229:1769, 1974.

73. Sklaroff, D. M. The uptake of radioactive rubidium Ru[86] by breast tumors. *A.J.R.* 79:994, 1958.

74. Sodee, D. B., Renner, R. R., and DiStefano, B. Photoscanning localization of tumor utilizing chlormerodrin mercury-197. *Radiology* 84:873, 1965.

75. Sugarbaker, P. H., Beard, J. O., and Drum, D. E. Detection of hepatic metastases from cancer of the breast. *Am. J. Surg.* 133:531, 1977.

76. Tofe, A. J., Francis, M. D., and Harvey, W. J. Correlation of neoplasms with incidence and localization of skeletal metastases: An analysis of 1,355 diphosphonate bone scans. *J. Nucl. Med.* 16:986, 1975.

77. Villarreal, R. L., Parkey, R. W., and Bonte, F. J. Experimental pertechnetate mammography. *Radiology* 111:657, 1974.

78. Weinraub, J. M., Rosenberg, R., and Irwin, G. A. L. ^{99m}Tc-polyphosphate in differential diagnosis of breast masses (abstract). *J. Nucl. Med.* 16:581, 1975.

79. Weissmann, H. S., Frank, M., Rosenblatt, R., et al. Cholescintigraphy, ultrasonography, and computerized tomography in the evaluation of biliary tract disorders. *Sem. Nucl. Med.* 9:22, 1979.

80. Witek, J. T., and Spencer, R. P. Scan evidence of decrease in size of intrahepatic tumors after chemotherapy. *Gastroenterology* 67:516, 1974.

Richard E. Wilson

8. Surgery for Breast Cancer

Philosophy of Primary Therapy

The surgeon treating primary breast cancer has three goals. The first is to control primary disease and prevent local recurrence; the second is to eradicate the source of continuing metastases; and the third is to permit the best possible rehabilitation on physical and psychological bases. Unfortunately, the disease must be treated in prospect, and the exact extent of the lesion is not known until after resection. The risk of distant metastases is always present, but the presence of local recurrence usually indicates that the disease was too far advanced for the form of treatment that was carried out. More sophisticated techniques for identifying micrometastases are on the horizon and the selection process for patients will improve progressively, but, nonetheless, the need for adequate primary therapy is of critical importance. A study at Guy's Hospital [1] in which only moderate-dose radiation plus partial mastectomy was utilized as a mode of therapy has demonstrated conclusively that, if nothing else, inadequate primary therapy results in a higher local recurrence rate for both stage I and stage II disease. There was also a higher mortality when stage II disease was not adequately treated.

An important and new component of the philosophy of primary therapy is the concept that initial treatment serves to identify the extent of disease, thus making selection of patients for appropriate adjuvant therapy more accurate. Naturally this presupposes that adjuvant therapy is of value in altering the recurrence of disease and survival of patients after primary treatment. These factors will be discussed at a later point, but the possibility of providing adjuvant therapy, such as chemotherapy, radiotherapy, or immunotherapy exists at the present time. The data obtained from the specimen at the time of primary treatment served to help select the best presently available adjuvant treatment.

Criteria for Primary Surgical Treatment

The decisions on primary treatment of breast cancer are based on the determination of whether or not the disease is localized to the breast and axillary nodes. While it is recognized that it takes several years for breast cancer to develop into a palpable lesion (greater than 1 cm in diameter) and with cancer cells most likely circulating in the bloodstream and lymphatics, there is no way of documenting the presence of micrometastases by presently available techniques. Thus, the determination of the presence of micrometastases represents the limit for exclusion of patients whose lesions are resectable for cure. The workup of a patient with primary breast cancer includes evaluation of the major sites of potential metastases; that is, the lungs, bones, liver, and regional soft tissue. All of these studies are built into the TNM staging (see pp. 53–55), which is primarily concerned with summarizing the local, regional, and distant extent of disease.

A chest x-ray is adequate for an initial workup. If there is any question of disease, whole lung tomography should be obtained. The complete blood count is a useful way of checking bone marrow function; the presence of either abnormal cells on smear or unexplained anemia or thrombocytopenia warrants further investigation of the bone marrow. Liver function tests measuring alkaline phosphatase, lactate dehydrogenase (LDH), and serum glutamic-oxaloacetic transaminase (SGOT) are probably more accurate as screening tests than are liver scans. Liver scans should be obtained for anyone with abnormal liver function tests but otherwise can be omitted.

A bone scan is the most efficient method of identifying occult metastases. Any positive bone scan should be accompanied by x-rays to rule out benign skeletal disease. If questionable, the bone may be biopsied to prove that any positive bone scan is indeed metastatic disease, since the therapy becomes entirely different under these circumstances. A recent study from the Peter Bent Brigham Hospital indicates that bone scans are most accurate in patients with T2 and T3 lesions and are rarely of value in patients with small lesions of the T1 variety [9]. Likewise, occult bone metastases correlate with positive lymph nodes but not quite as well as with lesion size. Certainly a bone scan should be obtained on any patient with proved carcinoma of the breast after mastectomy, if not before, as a baseline for further management.

Once the TNM staging has been completed for a given patient, then the decision can be made as to whether or not a lesion is resectable. Patients with T3b, T4, N2, or N3 disease should not be considered as candidates for primary curative resection, since the risk of metastases already occurring is too high and the potential for inadequate control of chest wall disease is too great to justify this type of operative management. Women with such advanced local disease, but without distant metastases, should have radiation therapy to the primary lesion. A recent publication from the Peter Bent Brigham Hospital that revealed the results of treatment of patients with locally inoperable disease has demonstrated the advantage of adding systemic therapy to radiation therapy, as compared to use of radiation therapy alone [12]. Unfortunately, because this was a small series without prospective randomization, the assumptions derived from this study are only to be considered presumptive.

An important consideration for the future will be whether estrogen receptor positive tumors in patients with unresectable local lesions should be treated with either hormone alteration or chemotherapy in addition to breast radiation [6, 8].

Surgical Options

The surgical options range from simple removal of the mass to the most extensive procedure, the extended radical mastectomy. These techniques have developed over many years and have been used by a variety of surgeons, each with his or her own particular bias. The historical progression from simple removal of the malignant lump, during the middle half of the nineteenth century, to Halsted's radical mastectomy must be recognized as a demonstration of our predecessors' struggles in trying to determine the best way to treat this most common of malignancies in the female. Naturally, many misconceptions have developed over the years about what factors were important in the development of the ideal operation.

Unfortunately, any resection of the breast leaves the patient with a deformity. The major question, which has by no means been answered, is whether or not the extent of local treatment affects survival rate. As already mentioned, inadequate local treatment is to be avoided, but variations in the extent of resection and the possible combination of resection with radiation in a multimodal approach are certainly present-day options in primary treatment. We must recognize that accurate evaluation of the results of primary therapy takes 10 to 15 years of follow-up, particularly in the most favorable patients, before any significant differences that could be the end result of alternative forms of therapy might become apparent. Any departure from the more standardized approach to treatment without adequate prospective randomized trials clearly showing that results are equivalent to alternative forms of treatment puts the patient at risk. This is the primary philosophy that most oncologic surgeons consider when selecting methods of treatment of primary breast cancer. Certainly the standard radical mastectomy as devised by Halsted and Meyer has a record of long-term patient survival, and results must be equal if another form of therapy is to be substituted for it. Only recently have sufficient prospective randomized trials been initiated, both in the United States and other countries to eventually answer this question. Until this happens, however, the conscience of the surgeon must dictate his decision as to how far he strays from this procedure.

Extended Radical Mastectomy

The extended radical mastectomy as popularized by J. Urban at Memorial Hospital and by Kaae and Johansen [7] includes the internal mammary chain of nodes with the primary specimen. These nodes are taken in continuity with a portion of intercostal fascia and chest wall. Most of its advocates will now only perform this for patients with medial or central lesions. There has been only minimal acceptance of this extended operation on the part of most surgeons throughout the world, since medial lesions behave much the same way as lateral lesions of the same stage and size.

Standard Radical Mastectomy

The standard radical mastectomy consists of a wide excision of the breast, with margins of skin extending at least 5 cm from the tumor. The skin flaps extend to the sternum medially, to the clavicle superiorly, to the rectus muscle inferiorly, and to the latissimus dorsi laterally. The axilla and its contents, as well as the pectoralis major and minor muscles, are included in the specimen; this has the advantage of including all of the interpectoral lymphatics and nodes as part of the resection. In general, the axillary dissection does not go above the axillary vein, so nodal tissue and fat in the vicinity of the brachial plexus are not necessarily included with the specimen. Whether or not skin grafts are required does not figure in the primary operative procedure. There is a major cosmetic defect when the pectoralis muscles are removed along with the specimen, the chest wall being more concave. Reconstruction is often less satisfactory after this form of mastectomy.

Modified Radical Mastectomy

This type of mastectomy consists of a total mastectomy performed in the same manner as the standard radical but the pectoralis musculature is left intact; the axillary lymph nodes are similarly removed. This procedure is performed either with or without removal of the pectoralis minor muscle. Some surgeons even split the pectoralis major to approach the highest axillary nodes; in this way, with adequate retraction, the interpectoral nodes and the highest axillary nodes usually can be removed satisfactorily. This operation has the advantage of accurate axillary staging and a full axillary dissection in continuity with the breast specimen, but it does not remove the penetrating lymphatics passing through the muscles. There is sufficient evidence from surgical resection for malignancy of the head and neck area and the extremities that lymphatic metastases are embolic and that it is not necessary to include all the lymphatic channels between the primary tumor and the drainage sites for adequate treatment. There are no data to demonstrate any difference in survival or recurrence of disease between these two forms of operative procedures.

The retained pectoralis muscles provide a better chest wall contour, which makes it easier to reconstruct the breast, since the prosthesis can be partially placed beneath the pectoralis muscle for greater mobility and less contracture. The modified radical mastectomy unquestionably has achieved great popularity among surgeons and is now performed by at least 90 percent of the practicing surgeons in the United States.

Simple Mastectomy

Simple mastectomy—a total mastectomy with adequate skin resection and full removal of all the breast tissue, including the nipple and the areola—is another form of treatment that has little to offer over the modified mastectomy. Full breast resection with its cosmetic consequences is carried out, yet there is no axillary dissection and therefore no adequate identification of lymphoid metastases. At present, there are no data to support the benefit of removal of nodes, even those involved with metastases. A clinical trial is presently being carried out by the National Surgical Adjuvant Breast Project (NSABP) to look at this very question [4]. Meaningful answers should be available in the next 5 to 10 years. For many years, particularly in Great Britain, the simple mastectomy was accompanied by irradiation to the axilla, supraclavicular area, chest wall, and internal mammary chain. In this way regional disease was treated with radiation, and local disease was treated surgically. McWhirter [10] in Edinburgh initiated this plan and his results have certainly been satisfactory, although it is impossible to determine the histologic lymph node status of patients treated in this manner.

Subcutaneous Mastectomy

The subcutaneous mastectomy is a procedure that removes all of the breast tissue from within the skin envelope of the breast, usually from either a submammary or a radial incision; the nipple is not removed. This procedure is not an adequate operation for invasive malignancy. The main advantage is skin preservation, so that complete restoration of the breast contour can be carried out during reconstruction, the result of which, cosmetically, can be identical to the still-existing breast. This procedure is best suited for patients with in situ carcinomas in which there is no invasion but the entire breast is at risk for subsequent spread. The operation is frequently performed bilaterally. The nipple can be preserved and carefully followed without any significant risk. The main concern of the surgeon must be complete removal of breast tissue, which requires experience and skill but can be accomplished successfully.

Partial Mastectomy

A partial mastectomy is any operation less than a total mastectomy; it ranges from hemi-mastectomy to simple removal of the lump (lumpectomy). The size of the primary tumor and its location and the breast contour determine the efficacy of this procedure. It is not always possible to totally remove the malignant tumor with a lumpectomy procedure since it may have broad extensions into the surrounding tissue. This is particularly true if the nodule is of large size. The partial mastectomy is most suited for small lesions that are amenable to added x-ray therapy. It has been the type of treatment advocated as a means of preserving the breast shape after treatment.

Results of Surgical Management as Primary Treatment

The National Surgical Adjuvant Breast Project has studied patients with clinically negative or positive nodes in two separate trials. The first, which reported on patients with clinically negative nodes, compared standard radical mastectomy to total mastectomy plus irradiation and total mastectomy alone. In the second, dealing with patients with clinically positive nodes, standard radical mastectomy was compared to total mastectomy and radiation. The data, as reported in 1977, included an approximately 36-month mean follow-up and showed life table projections extending to 42 months. In the patients with clinically negative nodes, 354 underwent radical mastectomy, with 87 percent survival; 282 underwent total mastectomy plus radiation, with 91 percent survival; and 344 had total mastectomy, with 86 percent survival. In the second group, 277 patients had radical mastectomy, with 73 percent survival; while 224 patients had total mastectomy with irradiation, with a 74 percent survival. Local recurrence was markedly reduced in these two groups having radiotherapy, as expected. Regional recurrence was not particularly altered, however, nor was the incidence of distant metastases. The percent of treatment failures in those with radical mastectomy was 20.9 percent; with mastectomy plus radiation, 19.1 percent; and with total mastectomy alone, 23.8 percent. Patients with clinically positive nodes having radical mastectomy showed a 37.9 percent treatment failure rate, while those with total mastectomy and radiation had a 38.4 percent failure rate. Obviously, then, there are no differences within the specific protocols for each of the two trials. If these data continue to hold for 10 years, they will be particularly valuable studies and will go a long way toward settling some of the issues regarding appropriate surgical management.

There are additional trials of importance. One of them, being carried out in Milan, compares patients with T1 N0 disease [13]. In these women, one treatment protocol is quadrant resection of the breast, including the lesion and axillary dissection, either en bloc or separate, depending on the location of the primary. This procedure is then combined with radiation therapy to the breast. Patients with positive nodes recieve cyclophosphamide, methotrexate, and 5-fluorouracil for 1 year. The other treatment protocol is the standard radical mastectomy. In this series of 331 patients, about one quarter were found to have histologically positive axillary nodes that were clinically thought to be negative. Of the 331 patients, 167 underwent radical mastectomy and 164 had the more conservative procedure with radiation. Although it is still too early to evaluate the results, to date there are no differences between the groups in either deaths or recurrences.

Several other clinical trials have been reported in the recent past [3, 5]. They have also shown that results of conservative therapy without pectoral muscle removal have been equivalent to those of radical mastectomy and that results of limited axillary node sampling has not been appreciably different from those with en bloc axillary dissection. The major unanswered questions in reviewing results of various surgical treatments for primary breast cancer are related to long-term survival for limited resections (10-plus years) and whether or not tumor-bearing lymph nodes that are left in situ carry a greater risk for eventual metastases and mortality than if they are removed with the breast.

There are several features of the primary lesion that are now recognized as being important in determining results of therapy. Any prospective randomized trial must appropriately stratify for these various features in order for there to be adequate comparison of data between groups. The stage, on both a clinical and histologic basis, is essential. The stage is a combination of tumor size and lymph node status. Histologic proof of metastatic involvement of the lymph nodes and the size of the lesion are both important determinants, whereas the clinical lymph node stage is of no consequence if it is incorrect. In other words, histologic stage II is the critical feature, not clinical stage I, in a patient who turns out to have microscopically involved lymph nodes. Patients with lesions greater than 2 cm (T2) have a worse prognosis than those with lesions smaller than 2 cm, while those with lesions greater than 5 cm are definitely at greater risk for recurrence.

The accurate histologic stage must be the final criterion for comparison of treatment groups. The pathologist must be skilled in identifying multifocal primary cancers, the tumor margins, the size of the lesion, and the presence and number of involved nodes. More than four involved nodes in the axilla clearly carries a greater risk than one to three involved lymph nodes. The presence of reactive hyperplasia in lymph nodes is considered important and a good prognostic sign by some investigators. The distribution of nodal metastases between nodes in the apex of the axilla, in the middle third, and in nodes closest to the breast must be delineated. In general, the axillary nodes are divided into these three groups, and apical axillary involvement carries a worse prognosis than the other two. The presence of the more favorable lesions such as adenoid cystic, cribriform, and medullary carcinomas must be identified.

The tumor margins within the breast are critical. This is particularly true for the posterior aspect adjacent to muscle. When the surgeon is performing a mastectomy and tumor seems to be posteriorly placed in the breast, it is essential that some of the underlying muscle be resected with the specimen. The decision as to whether or not radiation therapy should be added to mastectomy may, on occasion, depend on the posterior margin of the resection. Likewise, the skin margins and the extent of tumor into the skin overlying the breast tissue are important criteria for prognosis. Skin involvement always indicates true metastases. The presence of inflammatory carcinoma with both clinical evidence of inflammation and tumor-induced cellulitis with histologic demonstration of intralymphatic skin involvement is an important factor influencing survival. The age and menopausal status of the patient may be of prognostic value. Although breast cancer is more common after the menopause, the disease has always seemed to be somewhat more aggressive in the younger patient. Certainly it is often in a more advanced stage at the time of diagnosis in young women, primarily because of delay in diagnosis. There is no proof, however, from end-result reporting at the NCI [11], that stage for stage, younger patients have any different results. Without question, the menopausal status of the patient can affect response to adjuvant chemotherapy, younger patients responding more favorably.

Quantity of estrogen receptor protein in the malignant tumor may be an important prognostic factor. Recently a group from the University of Chicago [2] demonstrated that not only is the estrogen receptor protein a valuable predictor of response for hormonal alteration after metastatic disease has developed, but also it is a predictor of the total course of the patient with primary breast cancer. Those patients who are estrogen receptor positive have a longer disease-free interval, a lower recurrence rate, and a better survival rate than those without receptors present in the tumor. These are relatively preliminary concepts, but they may have some importance in better understanding the overall results of primary treatment.

Surgical Management of Local Metastatic Disease

Since the biologic concept of primary breast cancer generally is that it is a systemic disease, it is particularly important to understand that the management of local recurrence of breast cancer must be viewed from the standpoint of regional and systemic therapy. Approximately 90 percent of patients who develop local recurrence already have metastatic disease or their metastases become clinically detectable within 6 months. Sir J. Bruce has shown that 86 percent of patients who develop recurrence tend to do so within the first 5 years, and, in fact, the great majority have manifested their recurrence in the first 3 years. The term *local recurrence* is usually applied to metastases developing either on the chest wall itself following mastectomy or primary radiation or in the regional lymph nodes. These are the axillary, supraclavicular, and internal mammary nodes on the ipsilateral side of the primary tumor. Metastatic disease arising in the contralateral nodal groups is considered distant, as is spread to the opposite breast.

The disease-free interval represents the time span between the primary treatment of the breast cancer and the first clinical identification of either local or distant metastases. Involvement of the chest wall may either be intradermal or subcutaneous. Subcutaneous nodules can be solitary and are the only type of local recurrence that does not necessarily represent distant disease. The nodules represent small nests of tumor cells in residual breast tissue that was not adequately excised or in the subcutaneous fat that was contiguous with the breast at the time of the original operation. The usual pattern, however, is for there to be simultaneous development of distant and local recurrence, providing a gross indication of major alterations of host-tumor relationships. These nests of tumor cells most likely were present since the time of original treatment; yet, for them to suddenly become clinically apparent 2 or more years after the original operation requires that there be a change in the growth characteristics.

The patterns of metastatic disease in breast cancer generally tend to fall into three categories. The first of these is soft tissue disease involving local and regional recurrence, including any site on the chest wall, supraclavicular area, brachial plexus, or opposite breast. The second type of metastatic pattern is skeletal, and the third form is visceral, including lung, pleura, liver, and brain.

Whenever local recurrence has been identified, it is essential to thoroughly investigate all other potential sites of metastases before any treatment is instituted for apparent limited disease. While metastatic disease has a greater probability of occurring in patients with stage II or stage III disease than in those with stage I disease, local recurrence is most frequently associated with a more advanced lesion within the breast itself (T3 and T4). Typical findings for higher risk of local recurrence are edema of the skin, inflammatory lesions of the breast, ulceration and fixation of the skin, and larger-sized lesions.

As surgeons learn to be more selective about which patients should have primary surgical management and which ones are candidates for systemic treatment, less local recurrence will be seen. It is generally accepted that the presence of local recurrence usually indicates that the local disease in the original breast was too far advanced for local resection to have been attempted. Although the presence of positive axillary nodes is associated with a higher incidence of local recurrence, it has been the usual experience that T3 and T4 lesions are the ones most likely to demonstrate chest wall metastases.

As with any malignancy, the development of a nodule, either intradermally or subcutaneously, demands a biopsy. This can usually be performed under local anesthesia on an outpatient basis. Any malignant tissue that is found should be studied for estrogen receptor protein. Lymph nodes that might be involved should also be studied for estrogen receptor activity, since the determination of the estrogen receptor protein in metastatic lesions is possibly more valid for directing therapy of metastatic disease than is the identification of estrogen receptor protein in the original primary breast cancer.

Once the recurrent nodule has been biopsied and the presence of metastatic breast cancer is confirmed, the usual therapy is to radiate the chest wall and the regional lymph nodes. In all likelihood, this form of recurrence will occur in patients who have not had prior radiation. If they have had prior radiation, this treatment option is not usually available.

Important decisions have to be made as to whether the treatment for regional or local recurrence should be only local or systemic in nature. Systemic metastases are sought for by the usual clinical studies, including bone scan, liver scan, liver function tests, diagnostic radiography, and a thorough physical examination. Generally, for recurrence only on the chest wall, particularly for the subcutaneous nodule, excisional biopsy and radiation suffice until there is proven evidence of distant disease. For regional nodal involvement other than axillary, systemic therapy is more frequently the treatment of choice. Axillary nodal metastases, once biopsied, should not be treated by any radical surgery. It is preferable to perform a biopsy to identify recurrence and to study the tissue for estrogen receptor protein, to be followed by radiation therapy to the local region for good control. If other disease is present in a distant location, it is not necessary to use radiation locally unless there are local symptoms that do not respond to systemic therapy.

If a patient's original surgical treatment was a partial mastectomy, it can be converted to a total mastectomy if recurrence occurs within the breast. This is independent of additional radiation. Determining the extent of involvement throughout the rest of the breast and the presence of disease in the lymph nodes in the axilla will help determine the subsequent management of the patient. Disease that remains localized to the breast with or without positive axillary nodes, even in a patient who has previously undergone irradiation, can still be treated as local disease if a thorough workup for metastases is negative. The primary approach for all patients presenting with local recurrence, however, is to search for distant disease and to utilize systemic therapy if distant metastases exist. Even when distant metastases are not found, careful and frequent observation should be used to reevaluate the patient for this possibility. The patient must be made particularly aware of the need for close follow-up evaluation.

Surgical Management After Failure of Primary Radiation Therapy

Fortunately recurrence after primary radiation therapy has not been frequent. There has been sufficient evidence that radiation therapy following mastectomy will reduce the incidence of chest wall and regional recurrence, so one of the major advantages of primary radiation therapy should conceivably be a low incidence of regional and local recurrence. This has been apparent in the results of the NSABP trial to date. The use of chemotherapy following radiation in histologic stage II patients (when the axilla has been explored and biopsied) may reduce the incidence of local recurrence in these patients even further. When recurrence does occur after primary radiation therapy, however, it is difficult to manage.

The heavily radiated breast, with the irradiation often boosted with local radiation implants, frequently cannot receive any further radiation therapy. Simple mastectomy is the treatment of choice for patients who have recurrences in the breast after radiation therapy, although skin coverage is always a technical problem. The development of flaps for resection of the breast tissue may be difficult because of compromised vascular supply. When the actual blood supply of any portion of the skin is difficult to define, then flap viability is always in question. Therefore, minimal flap formation after radiation therapy is the rule, with either a planned preparation for a pedicle graft or use of local skin grafts.

There may be sepsis in the breast with recurrent cancer, particularly if the skin overlying the tumor breaks down. This is, unfortunately, a common occurrence. There may also be underlying bone and lung damage from radiation therapy, especially in patients treated in the past with orthovoltage technique. It may be necessary to perform the chest wall coverage in several stages. Pedicle flaps can be developed from the abdomen, the other breast, or the back to provide full thickness coverage of the defect with a fat pad. Another possibility is to bring the omentum from the abdomen across the costal margin into the defect and apply skin grafts directly to this vascular surface. Each patient presenting with recurrence after irradiation poses individual and unique problems requiring careful judgment decisions for management.

Planning for Reconstruction When Performing Primary Procedures

The major problems associated with reconstruction have to do with development of the skin flaps and the provision of space for the prosthesis. The eventual success of and satisfaction with a prosthesis depends on its prolonged softness and pliability. If the skin is too taut or infection and extensive fibrosis intervene, the prosthesis will have to be removed. When reconstruction is considered, a horizontal incision for the mastectomy provides a better result. Because the blood supply then is more likely to be on a horizontal basis from the intercostal arteries, the upper and lower flaps would be more likely to be well vascularized. This incision does not extend on the chest wall above or to the superior surface of the prosthesis and is therefore much more acceptable. When possible, the skin grafts should not be used, as they may interfere with subsequent dissection of the chest wall flaps for placement of the prosthesis. Although the grafts do not have the expansile capability that normal skin has, if they are necessary, they should be as thick as possible. Postoperative irradiation may reduce the blood supply to the skin flaps and certainly should be done only after careful consideration.

Reconstruction should not be done for 6 to 12 months after mastectomy. This gives the surgeon time to determine what the maximum skin mobility will be and also allows insight into the risks for recurrent cancer. The major reason for the delay is to allow the skin to become pliable so that healing is more complete and fibrosis is least likely to occur. The reconstructive surgery can be done very expeditiously during a short hospital admission or even on an outpatient basis.

Preservation of the nipple may be unwise. Breast cancer recurrence within the transplanted nipple has been reported. The nipple consists of the orifices of all the major breast ducts and as such is in contact with the entire breast. In women with invasive breast cancer, implantation of the nipple in the groin runs the risk of reimplanting those cells on the patient's chest wall rather than eliminating them from the host. The nipple, even when placed back on the reconstructed breast, will have no sensation. It can be reconstructed instead from the opposite breast or labia or a nipple may be tattooed on the skin of the new breast mound with excellent results.

One of the advantages of performing subcutaneous mastectomy in the breast opposite to the cancerous one is the ease of placing symmetric bilateral prostheses. This is usually preferred to any reduction mammoplasty for the other breast since the latter tends to distort the breast tissue and makes a follow-up more difficult.

General Results of Reconstruction

Breast reconstruction should be offered to any woman undergoing mastectomy. Preferably this should be brought up at the time of the first visit when the mass in the breast is identified. It certainly should be stressed during the hospital course, and, if possible, the plastic surgeon who might perform such a reconstruction should see the patient at the time of her primary mastectomy.

Not all women are interested in having reconstruction of the breast, especially when results may be somewhat uncertain. Healing can vary from patient to patient, and the contracture of scar around the prosthesis can make the result less satisfactory. In general, it is the younger woman and the woman who is active in sports and leads a busy and vigorous life who is the most interested in reconstruction. It allows her to be free of the need for an external prosthesis and its attendant psychological and logistic problems. Insertion of a prosthesis is a simple and brief procedure and, in most cases, utilizes a portion of the previous mastectomy scar. The prosthesis does not interfere with careful follow-up examination of the skin and subcutaneous fat, which is the location of virtually all local chest wall recurrence. The decision as to whether the prosthesis should be placed in the subpectoral position depends on local factors and may result in differences in fibrosis and skin mobility.

A major advantage to breast reconstruction is to make the concept of mastectomy more acceptable, thus resulting in less delay. Unquestionably, breast reconstruction must assume its proper place in the rehabilitation of the mastectomy patient.

References

1. Atkins, H., Bulbrook, R. D., Falconer, M. A., et al. Ten years experience of steroid assays in the management of breast cancer. *Lancet* 2:1255, 1968.
2. Block, G. E., Ellis, R. S., DeSombre, E., and Jensen, E. Correlation of estrophilin content of primary mammary cancer to eventual endocrine treatment. *Ann. Surg.* 188:372, 1978.
3. Brinkley, D., and Haybittle, J. L. The treatment of stage II carcinoma of the female breast. *Lancet* 2:291, 1966.
4. Fisher, B., Montague, E., Redmond, C., et al. Comparison of radical mastectomy with alternative treatments for primary breast cancer: A first report of results from a prospective randomized clinical trial. *Cancer* 39:2827, 1977.
5. Forrest, A. P. M. Conservative local treatment of breast cancer. *Cancer* 39:2813, 1977.
6. Jensen, E. V., Block, G. E., Smith, S., et al. Estrogen receptors and breast cancer response to adrenalectomy. Prediction of response in breast cancer therapy. National Cancer Institute Monograph. Washington, D.C.: U.S. Government Printing Office, 1971. P. 34.
7. Kaae, S., and Johansen, H. Simple mastectomy plus postoperative irradiation by the method of McWhirter for mammary carcinoma. *Ann. Surg.* 179:895, 1969.
8. McGuire, W. L., Horwitz, K. B., Pearson, O. H., and Segaloff, A. Current status of estrogen and progesterone receptors in breast cancer. *Cancer* 39:2934, 1977.
9. McNeil, B. J., Pace, P. D., Gray, E. B., et al. Preoperative and followup bone scans in patients with operable breast cancer. *Surg. Gynecol. Obstet.* 147:745, 1978.
10. McWhirter, R. The value of simple mastectomy and radiotherapy in the treatment of cancer of the breast. *Br. J. Radiol.* 21:599, 1948.
11. National Cancer Institute. Cancer Patient Survival. Report No. 5; U.S. Department of Health, Education and Welfare, Public Health Service, National Institutes of Health. Washington, D.C.: U.S. Government Printing Office, 1976. P. 157.
12. Osteen, R. T., Chaffey, J. T., Moore, F. D., and Wilson, R. E. An aggressive multimodality approach to locally advanced carcinoma of the breast. *Surg. Gynecol. Obstet.* 147:75, 1978.
13. Veronesi, U., Banfi, A., Saccozzi, R., et al. Conservative treatment of breast cancer: A trial in progress at the Cancer Institute of Milan. *Cancer* 39(Suppl. 6):2822, 1977.

Jay R. Harris
Martin B. Levene
Samuel Hellman

9. Radiotherapy and Breast Carcinoma

Radiation therapy, like surgery, is a form of local and regional treatment for carcinoma of the breast. Its purpose is to provide local and regional tumor control with eradication of cancer in the breast and draining lymph node areas. Radiation therapy has been used traditionally as a treatment after mastectomy in cases of early cancer in order to provide greater assurance of local tumor control and in locally treating advanced cancers that are poorly managed by mastectomy. More recently, radiation therapy has been used as an alternative to mastectomy in early breast cancer in order to obtain local and regional control while preserving the breast [8]. In this chapter, we will present our current indications for radiation therapy in the local management of breast cancer and describe our method of treatment. At the present time there are encouraging preliminary reports on various forms of treatment for breast cancer [1]. The indications for surgery, radiation therapy, and adjuvant systemic therapy in primary management are likely to evolve as additional data become available.

Basic Principles of Clinical Radiation Therapy

An idealized illustration of the relationship of local tumor control and complications to radiation dose is found in Figure 9-1. While both local tumor control and complications have a sigmoid relationship to dose, the complication curve is displaced to the right of the tumor control curve. If these curves are significantly separated, the chance for an uncomplicated cure is high. On the other hand, if the curves are superimposable, the chance for an uncomplicated cure is low. The degree of separation of these curves is the measure of the therapeutic gain possible with radiation treatment. Several factors affecting the therapeutic gain have been identified, including tumor cell type, amount of normal tissue irradiated, volume of radiation, time-

215

dose relationships of the radiation therapy, and bulk of tumor treated. Different tumor cell types respond to variable degrees of local control by radiation. Seminomas and lymphomas are among the most radiocurable tumors, while soft tissue sarcomas and glioblastoma multiforme are among the most refractory. Breast cancers are in an intermediate position, being similar to squamous cell carcinomas of the head and neck region and of the uterine cervix.

Normal tissues similarly have variable degrees of sensitivity to the effects of radiation. Ovarian and testicular reproductive functions are permanently abolished by as small a dose as 1500 rads over 2 weeks. In contrast, portions of the vaginal mucosa and ureters can receive doses as great as 10,000 rads over 8 weeks without significant functional deficits. The critical normal tissues associated with breast cancer radiation are the chest wall, lung, heart, and bone marrow.

A third factor affecting therapeutic gain is the volume of irradiated tissue. This factor is of great importance, since the likelihood of a complication for a given normal tissue is critically dependent on the volume of tissue irradiated. For example, small portions of the lung can receive as much as 5000 to 6000 rads over 7 weeks without clinically apparent deficit, while exposing the entire lung to 2000 rads over 2 weeks will frequently result in serious radiation pneumonitis. The volume of bone marrow irradiated in treating carcinoma of the breast represents less than 5 percent of the total marrow, and blood count problems related to this treatment are rare. The volume of lung and heart that is irradiated is highly dependent on the technique of treatment. The use of techniques that minimize exposure to these normal tissues is important to ensure that occurrences of radiation pneumonitis and pericarditis are uncommon.

The time-dose relationships of radiation therapy refer to the number of treatments given and the elapsed time between the initiation and completion of these treatments. Clinical experience has demonstrated that the therapeutic gain is improved by fractionation of the radiation treatments. This fractionation over an extended period of time provides greater recovery of the normal tissues over the tumor. In most tumors the best results are achieved when a daily dose of 180 to 200 rads is used. The total dose required to obtain local tumor control is critically dependent on the bulk of the tumor treated. For breast cancer,

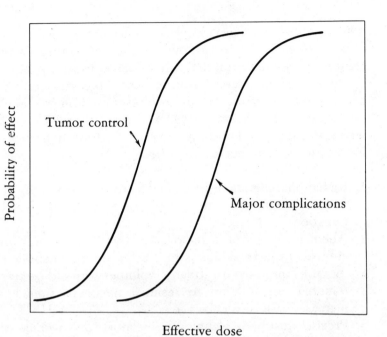

Figure 9–1. Relationship of local tumor control and major complications to radiation dose.

4500 to 5000 rads over 5 weeks is sufficient for the eradication of microscopic amounts of tumor, while doses of 6000 rads or greater are required for clinically palpable disease.

Modern radiotherapeutic management of breast cancer is based on the implementation of this dose-response principle in order to maximize the chances for local tumor control while minimizing the likelihood of complications. The following guidelines for treatment have been established.

1. Radiation treatment is facilitated by resection of bulky tumor masses, leaving only microscopic disease to be eradicated by radiation.
2. Adequate doses of radiation are required for local tumor control. In general this is best achieved by combining external beam radiation to large volumes with radioactive interstitial implantation to residual tumor or sites having increased risk of recurrence.
3. Precise treatment planning is essential for coverage of all potentially involved areas, maximal sparing of normal tissue, and the avoidance of overlapping fields.

Primary Radiation Therapy for Stage I and II Carcinoma of the Breast

While mastectomy has been shown to be an effective means of obtaining local control in up to 90 percent of patients with early breast cancer, this form of surgery has been a harsh physical and emotional experience for many women. For this reason, physicians caring for women with breast cancer have sought equally effective, but less deforming, methods of local treatment. In this country, attention recently has been directed to the use of primary radiation therapy as an alternative to mastectomy.

The use of radiation therapy has been based on three principal factors. First, primary radiation therapy has been used as sole treatment for a variety of other early human cancers as a means of preserving form and function in preference to surgery [5]. These include early malignancies of the larynx, mouth, throat, prostate, penis, and skin, as well as some brain tumors and soft tissue sarcomas. In all such cases, primary radiation therapy provides equivalent local control rates; and, since it is less deforming, it is frequently the treatment of choice. The use of primary radiation therapy for early breast cancer therefore has a precedent in other human cancers. Second, radiation therapy performed after mastectomy for breast cancer has clearly produced a drastic reduction in the incidence of local and regional recurrences. A logical extension of the observation that moderate doses of radiation can eradicate microscopic amounts of breast cancer is to combine total excisional biopsy of the primary tumor mass with postoperative radiation for eradication of microscopic deposits of tumor. This combination of conservative surgery and moderate doses of radiation therapy constitutes the primary radiation therapy treatment plan. Third, while primary radiation therapy has been used only recently in this country, results of long-term use of this form of treatment are available from other countries, particularly Canada [12], Finland [11], and France [13, 15], and have shown results comparable to mastectomy.

On the basis of these three factors, a large number of institutions in this country in recent years have treated women with early breast cancer with primary radiation therapy. The experience at our institution is representative of these recent studies and illustrates that primary radiation therapy can achieve local control rates comparable to those seen with mastectomy and still maintain good to excellent cosmetic results for the large majority of patients (Fig. 9-2) [9, 10]. Five-year survival of these patients also appears to be comparable to that of surgically treated patients, but further follow-up is required because of the long natural history of this disease.

In both the biopsy procedure and radiation therapy, results stress the importance of the technical details in achieving the dual objectives of local control and good cosmetic results. Treatment begins with the biopsy procedure. Local control appears to be improved in those patients undergoing excisional biopsy as opposed to patients having less than excisional biopsies. On the other hand, in some patients the cosmetic result was ruined by excessively wide resections. We recommend a total gross excision of the primary tumor.

The size and location of the biopsy incision are also important; small unobtrusive incisions give the best cosmetic results. When feasible, circumareolar or inframammary incisions are

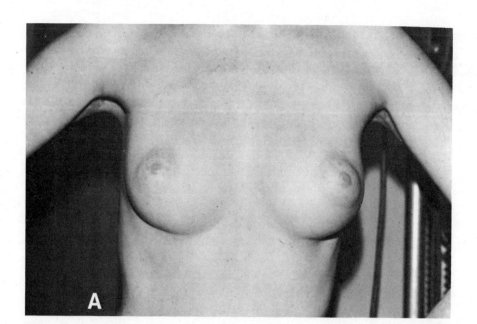

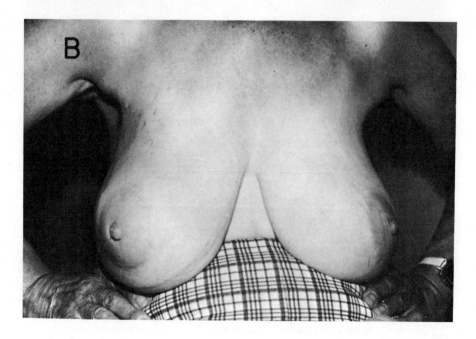

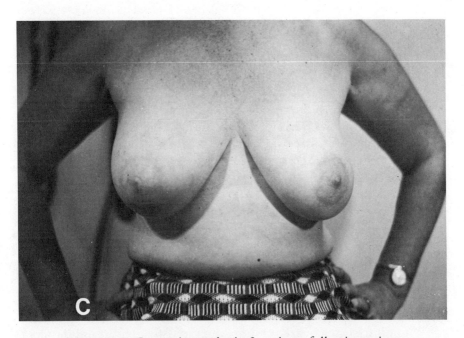

Figure 9–2. Cosmetic results in 3 patients following primary radiation therapy. A. This patient had a T1 N0 carcinoma of the right breast. She underwent excisional biopsy followed by 5000 rads in 25 fractions. The photograph was taken 3 years and 10 months from the end of treatment. B. This patient had a T2 N0 carcinoma of the right breast and underwent excisional biopsy; she then received 5000 rads in 25 fractions, followed by interstitial implant of the primary tumor area for an additional 2000 rads. The photograph was taken 2 years and 10 months from the end of treatment. C. This woman had a T1 N0 carcinoma of the left breast. She underwent excisional biopsy followed by 5400 rads in 27 fractions. The photograph was taken 1 year and 4 months from the end of treatment.

preferred. Surgery in the form of axillary sampling also may be required. Here, too, the use of small, unobtrusive incisions and the avoidance of excessive dissection are recommended. At our institution, patients considered for adjuvant chemotherapy routinely undergo axillary sampling. The same guidelines of axillary node involvement used to determine the need for chemotherapy in patients undergoing mastectomy are used in patients undergoing axillary sampling and primary radiation therapy.

Radiation therapy is begun with external beam radiation. Patients are treated with a three-field technique consisting of opposed tangential fields to the breast, lower axilla, and internal mammary nodes, and an anterior field to the axillary apex and supraclavicular region. Prior to treatment, precise planning and setup of treatment fields is accomplished with the use of a simulator, which duplicates the geometry of the treatment machine but gives diagnostic radiographs. Care must be taken to avoid overlapping fields if previous irradiation has been administered (Fig. 9-3). (We have recently modified our technique to minimize such overlap.) Individual styrofoam head and shoulder casts are made to ensure reproducibility of patient setup from day to day.

Treatment is delivered with a 4 MeV linear accelerator. Supervoltage equipment of this kind produces relative sparing of the uppermost 1 to 2 mm of skin from radiation damage. As a result, the skin returns to its normal color and consistency following treatment. In the more advanced cases in which skin involvement is present or suspected, the skin sparing is circumvented by applying a layer of material called bolus on the skin during treatment; this material takes the place of the normally spared skin. In early cases, however, the uppermost layer of the skin is not at risk for tumor, and, since it will adversely affect the cosmetic result, the use of bolus may not be recommended.

Homogeneity of radiation dose throughout the tumor volume is important. While the likelihood of tumor control is primarily determined by the minimum tumor doses, complications are frequently determined by the maximum tumor dose. For this reason, excessive inhomogeneity of radiation doses is associated with an increased incidence of complications without an increase in tumor control. Because of the irregular contour

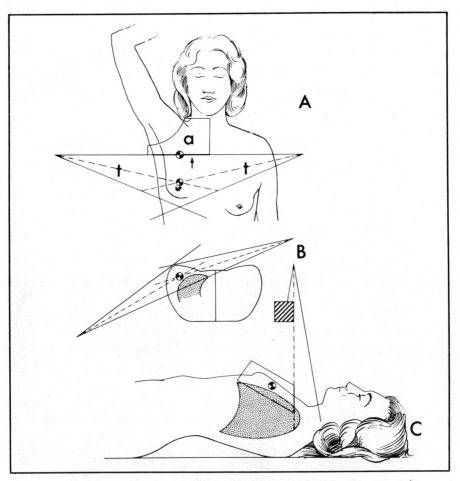

Figure 9–3. Field arrangement of external beam treatment of carcinoma of the breast. A. Coronal projection. The two almost opposing and isocentric tangential fields (t) treat the breast, internal mammary nodes, and lower axilla. The anterior field (a), with a humeral head block, irradiates the axillary apex and supraclavicular region. The heavy line between the anterior field and the tangents is referred to as the matchline (*small arrow*). The half-filled circle represents the isocenter. Note that the tangential fields are angled so that the superior borders coincide. B. Cross-sectional projection. This projection shows that, if properly angled, the deep edges of the tangential fields are coincident. C. Sagittal projection. The medial tangential and the anterior fields are shown in this view. Accurate matching in three dimensions is achieved by using a special blocking arrangement on the tangential fields (not explicitly shown) and a central axis block on the inferior portion of the anterior field (hatched section).

encompassed by the tangential fields, dose inhomogeneity in the breast is significant unless tissue compensators are used. We routinely use wedge-shaped filters as tissue compensators to correct for irregular contours and improve dose homogeneity in the tangential fields.

External beam treatment is given 5 days a week at 200 rads per day for a total of 5000 rads in 5 to $5\frac{1}{2}$ weeks. Each treatment takes approximately 20 minutes, with the majority of that time spent on patient setup. In general, treatments are very well tolerated, with most patients continuing to work during treatment. The chief complaints encountered during treatment are fatigue and skin irritation, both of which are seen toward the end of treatment. Nausea and vomiting are uncommon, and cranial alopecia does not occur. Following completion of external beam therapy, the patient is given a 2-week rest to allow healing of the skin reaction.

After the rest period, the patient is admitted to the hospital for an interstitial implant at the primary tumor site. Most frequently this procedure is performed under general anesthesia to facilitate the introduction of hollow plastic catheters in the prescribed geometric arrangement about the primary site. Following the patient's return to her room, radioactive material (iodine-192 at our institution) is passed into the catheter, providing radiation to the area at greatest risk. This form of radiation will only affect areas immediately adjacent to it, thus sparing normal structures nearby. Figure 9-4 illustrates the radiation dose distribution seen with interstitial implantation. The implant remains in place for 2 to 3 days. During this time patients are confined to their rooms but are up and about at liberty. Local recurrences are reduced by the use of interstitial implantation, and this procedure is now routinely performed after completion of external beam therapy.

At this time we find our results using primary radiation therapy highly encouraging. While mastectomy is still the traditional form of local treatment for carcinoma of the breast, we believe that primary radiation therapy is a reasonable alternative for women who have strong feelings about breast preservation. The current Joint Center for Radiation Therapy (JCRT) procedural guidelines for treating stage I and II carcinoma of the breast by primary radiation therapy are summarized in Table 9-1.

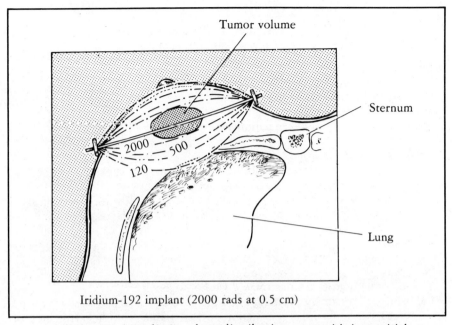

Iridium-192 implant (2000 rads at 0.5 cm)

Figure 9–4. Radiation dose distribution seen with interstitial implantation. In this illustration, 2000 rads is delivered to the tumor volume while nearby normal tissues receive normal minimal doses.

Table 9-1 Current JCRT Guidelines for Treatment of Stage I and II
Carcinoma of the Breast by Primary Radiation Therapy

Biopsy procedure
  Excisional biopsy
  Resection of small rim of normal breast tissue—not a wide local excision
  Small, unobtrusive incisions
  Sampling of axillary nodes in patients considered for adjuvant chemotherapy

Time/dose factors of radiation therapy
  Total external beam dose of 5000 rads over 5 to $5^1/_2$ weeks
  Fraction size: 200 rads per day, 5 days per week
  Interstitial implantation of the primary tumor site following external beam
    treatment for additional dose of 1500 to 2000 rads

Radiation therapy technique
  Supervoltage equipment
  No bolus
  Tissue compensators to maximize dose homogeneity
  Individualized treatment planning to ensure coverage of all potentially involved
    areas, with maximal sparing of normal tissue and the avoidance of
    overlapping fields

Postoperative Radiation in Stage I and II Carcinoma of the Breast

The incidence of local and regional recurrences following either
modified radical or radical mastectomy has been reported to be
10 to 25 percent [4, 6, 17]. Postoperative radiation has been
attempted in order to improve local and regional control of
recurrences and, perhaps, to improve survival. Results from a
number of studies now demonstrate, however, that, although
postoperative radiation significantly reduces this incidence of
local and regional recurrences, it does not improve survival for
treated patients as a whole [4, 17]. These results indicate that
survival for the majority of patients is predominantly determined by the presence of occult distant spread at the time of
mastectomy and not by the presence of residual local and regional tumor. Because most patients who have residual local
and regional tumor also have occult distant spread, postoperative radiation is not curative for these patients. It is now clear
that adjuvant systemic therapy, which is effective in eradicating
occult distant spread, is required to improve survival in the
majority of patients with regional disease. Nevertheless, there
do appear to be some patients in whom only residual local or
regional disease is present, disease that will metastasize if left

untreated. Recently attempts have been made to identify these subsets of patients who are likely to show a survival benefit from postoperative radiation. Current data suggests that two subsets of patients should receive such treatment: (1) those with medial or central primaries and positive axillary nodes, and (2) those with four or more positive nodes.

Postoperative radiation has a role apart from its effect on survival. Once manifest, local and regional recurrences are effectively treated in only 50 to 60 percent of patients [3, 19]. These recurrences frequently become the dominant factor in the lives of patients. For this reason, postoperative radiation is commonly recommended for patients in whom there is high risk of local and regional recurrence.

Future recommendations regarding postoperative radiation depend on the results obtained with adjuvant chemotherapy. If chemotherapy proves effective in eradicating both occult distant spread and residual local and regional tumor, postoperative radiation will not be required. If, as it now appears, chemotherapy is more effective in eradicating occult distant spread, postoperative radiation will play an even more important role in ensuring local and regional tumor control. The use of adjuvant radiation and chemotherapy is evolving and may change as more results become available.

At the present time, the role of postoperative radiation in premenopausal women is unclear, but it may well be added to the therapeutic regimen of patients in whom the risk of local and regional recurrence is high. Because studies to date have failed to indicate any benefit from adjuvant chemotherapy in postmenopausal women, postoperative radiation must assume a larger role in these patients. We recommend postoperative radiation for postmenopausal women who have medial or central primaries with positive axillary nodes, or postmenopausal women who have four or more positive axillary nodes, regardless of the primary site in the breast, or any patient in whom the risk of local and regional recurrence is high.

The results from our own institution are typical of those seen in other studies and clearly demonstrate the capability of postoperative radiation to reduce local and regional recurrences [18]. At our institution 352 patients treated with postoperative radiation following modified or conventional radical mastectomy were retrospectively analyzed. These patients were referred for treatment because of increased concern about local and regional recurrence. Seven percent of the entire group had histologically positive nodes. The overall recurrence rate after radiation therapy was 5 percent and the regional recurrence rate was 1 percent. These results are significantly less than would be expected from surgery alone.

The technique of postoperative radiation varies with the clinical situation. All patients are treated on a 4 MeV linear accelerator, but treatments are individually planned. In those patients in whom there is a significant risk of internal mammary node involvement, an internal mammary lymphoscintigram is performed prior to treatment planning. This study is used to identify the position of internal mammary nodes.

Treatment is delivered by means of three separate fields: opposed tangential fields to the chest wall and to the lower internal mammary nodes, and an anterior field to the axillary apex, supraclavicular nodes, and upper internal mammary nodes. It is our impression that treatment of internal mammary nodes by means of tangential fields is better tolerated than treatment by a direct anterior field, which inadvertently treats the mediastinal structures and is invariably associated with overlapping fields. The axillary region is not generally included in the treatment volume because recurrences in that region are rare following a full dissection, and the risk of lymphedema is increased with such treatment. The axillary region may be treated. If there is doubt that a full dissection has been performed, as in patients with a small number of nodes recovered at surgery, or in patients with heavy involvement of axillary nodes. The dose delivered is 4500 rads in 20 fractions over 5 weeks. This dose is the minimum dose to the tumor-bearing volume at a depth of 3 cm for the supraclavicular field. If more than 50 percent of the axillary nodes are positive, a large tumor dose may be considered. For patients receiving adjuvant chemotherapy, especially Adriamycin, doses are reduced by approximately 10 percent because of the known radiomimetic effects of such chemotherapeutic agents.

Primary Radiation Therapy for Stage III Carcinoma of the Breast

Stage III carcinoma of the breast includes a wide range of locally advanced cancers characterized by any of the following features.

1. Primary mass greater than 5 cm
2. Primary mass fixed to the skin or chest wall
3. Fixed axillary nodes
4. Supraclavicular node involvement

All of these features are associated with a high risk of occult distant spread and, therefore, a poor prognosis. In addition, local control of these cancers by the use of surgery alone is significantly less effective than it is for stage I and II cancers, with local failure rates ranging from 20 percent to 50 percent [7, 16]. As a result radiation therapy, either alone or in conjunction with surgery, has come to play a major treatment role in this stage of the disease.

Results from our institution have demonstrated that primary radiation therapy can be an effective means of obtaining local control for the large majority of patients with stage III cancers [2]. These results, however, stress the importance of using adequate doses of radiation. When local control was examined according to total dose delivered, in those patients receiving more than 6000 rads, the rate of local control was 78 percent as compared with 39 percent for patients receiving less than 6000 rads. As in the treatment of stage I and II cancers, total or near-total excisional biopsy and the use of interstitial implantation were both associated with improved local control.

Since stage III disease includes such a wide diversity of locally advanced tumors, a high degree of individualization is required in local treatment. For patients with operable stage III lesions with primary tumors greater than 5 cm with or without palpable axillary lymph nodes, surgery is commonly not recommended because of the surgeon's desire to avoid extensive surgery in patients with a poor prognosis. In this situation, excisional biopsy of the primary tumor and removal of enlarged axillary nodes is recommended. External beam radiation, 5000 rads over 5 weeks, is then delivered to the breast and draining lymph node areas, followed by an interstitial implant at the primary tumor site. In our experience, local control has been excellent in patients undergoing both excisional biopsy and interstitial implantation. A mastectomy is warranted in those patients in whom the primary tumor occupies the majority of the breast and in whom an excisional biopsy by itself would be disfiguring.

For patients who are inoperable because of the extent of the tumor in the breast or axilla, a minimal biopsy for histologic confirmation and hormone receptor studies is recommended. External beam radiation to 5000 rads over 5 weeks is then delivered, after which patients are reevaluated. If there has been such an excellent response to treatment that an adequate interstitial implant of the primary can be performed, external beam treatment is terminated and an implant is performed. If there has been a good response but an interstitial implant is not feasible, two more choices are available. One is to continue with external beam radiation, by means of a smaller field, to areas of gross disease to a total dose of approximately 6000 rads and then perform an interstitial implant. The other is to proceed with mastectomy if technically feasible at that point. Wound healing has not been a problem following a preoperative dose of 5000 rads.

Since most stage III patients develop distant metastases, there is a clear need for effective adjuvant systemic therapy. In our experience [2], patients with stage III breast cancer who received adjuvant cytotoxic systemic therapy have had an improved 4-year relapse-free survival rate when compared with similarly staged patients not receiving adjuvant therapy. These results suggest that adjuvant cytotoxic systemic therapy is effective in extending the relapse-free interval for treated patients and may eventually indicate an improved cure rate. In addition to this improvement in relapse-free survival, patients receiving adjuvant therapy also showed improved local tumor control. There were no local failures in the 20 patients who received adjuvant therapy and radiation doses greater than 6000 rads.

While patients with stage III cancers require both local and systemic treatment, the proper sequencing of these treatments is still a matter of controversy. We feel that local radiation therapy should be administered prior to or concomitantly with systemic therapy because of the limited tumor responses seen with the currently available drugs [14]. Because of this limited response and because the drugs themselves might increase host susceptibility to metastatic spread, the plan of treatment should include some initial local radiation therapy before the initiation of chemotherapy. This is done to prevent continuing metastatic spread from the primary tumor during the chemotherapy treatment. One possible exception is the patient who is estrogen receptor positive and being treated with hormonal therapy. In such a patient, because initial local treatment would obscure whether or not a response to hormonal treatment has been achieved, it is usually advisable to delay the start of local treatment until a response has been determined.

The use of concomitant local radiation and systemic chemotherapy must be done with care since normal tissue reactions are commonly greater than those seen with radiation alone, especially when Adriamycin is used. We commonly reduce radiation doses by 10 percent.

Treatment of Bone Metastases

The most common site of symptomatic metastases from carcinoma of the breast is bone, and the most frequently affected bones are the pelvis, spine, ribs, and femurs. Bone metastases are initially manifested by stiffness and dull aching in the involved areas and tend to progress slowly with time. If left untreated, these metastases can progress to pathologic fractures. Physical examination frequently reveals local tenderness of the affected areas, but otherwise may be entirely normal. Radiographic findings, too, commonly lag behind the onset of symptoms. When x-ray changes are present, they usually show an osteolytic pattern, although an osteoblastic pattern is not uncommon. A bone scan is sometimes a more sensitive test for metastatic spread but can also be negative in the presence of disease. Because of this lag between clinical involvement and x-ray findings, local palliative treatment may be delivered to areas of bone pain in the absence of radiographic abnormalities in patients with known metastatic disease in other sites.

Symptomatic bone metastases from carcinoma of the breast are treated well by local palliative radiation therapy. Radiation produces complete or nearly complete pain relief in the large majority of patients with these metastases. Since radiation therapy is local in its effect, this treatment is best suited for patients with limited disease. In patients with widespread symptomatic involvement, local palliative radiation to one or two sites usually fails to provide overall clinical improvement despite local pain relief. In this setting, systemic treatment is preferred. The response time is variable; some patients obtain pain relief after one or two treatments, while in others months pass before relief is achieved.

While palliative treatment requires great individualization, certain guidelines are available. When treatment of bone metastases is planned, adjacent sites should be considered. It is best to include whole sections of bone in the treated volume in order to avoid difficulties with inadequate therapy. For example, treatment ports that do not completely cover the femoral neck or head or the sacroiliac joints are to be avoided. Precise marking and record-keeping are essential to avoid unintentional overlapping of fields. In our institution all treatment ports are permanently identified on the patient's skin by small tattoo marks at the corners of the field. This is most important in treating the spine in order to avoid an excessive dose to the spinal cord. As a general rule, the dose guidelines for normal tissue tolerance are to be respected as in primary radical treatment. However, in certain instances in which metastatic disease has recurred in previously treated areas and irreversible damage due to this disease appears imminent, repeat courses of radiation therapy are sometimes recommended despite the increased risks of radiation injury.

The choice of radiation dose depends on the clinical situation. In the case of a patient who has had a long disease-free interval prior to developing a single painful metastasis, treatment would likely be carried to 4000 rads at 250 rads per day over 4 weeks. At the other extreme is a patient with severe localized rib pain but who has metastatic disease over a wide area and in whom death is impending; treatment in this case would likely be given in a single 1000 rad fraction. In between these extremes, varying fractionation schedules can be selected that are appropriate to the clinical situation. The goals of treatment are to prevent recurrence of symptoms in the treated area for the remainder of the patient's lifetime and to deliver the treatment in the fastest and least morbid way. Clinical judgment is required in selecting the best fractionation schedule for a given clinical situation.

Of particular concern in the treatment of bone metastases is the prevention and treatment of pathologic fractures. Pathologic fractures of the femur or humerus are not uncommon in patients with metastatic breast cancer. Routine skeletal x-rays or bone scans are recommended in these patients to detect large osteolytic lesions prior to fracture. If such lesions are noted, prophylactic radiation is indicated, even in the absence of symptoms. Once a pathologic fracture of a long bone has occurred, surgery is required for internal fixation and stabilization. Methyl methacrylate is commonly used to provide increased support. Radiation following surgery is indicated in all cases to prevent local recurrence of tumor.

Treatment of Spinal Cord Compression

Spinal cord compression is a relatively common complication seen in patients with metastatic breast cancer. Local radiation therapy plays a major role in the treatment of this complication, either alone or in conjunction with surgery. Patients with spinal cord compression present with spine pain, which may be followed by motor or sensory loss. Metastases to the conus medullaris and cauda equina are characterized by saddle anesthesia (loss of urethral, vaginal, and rectal sensation) as well as decreased control of micturition. While spine films are useful in the diagnosis, a myelogram is essential to determine the precise location of the compression. In most cases an extradural mass is seen, along with complete obstruction of flow of contrast material in the subarachnoid space. As a result of this obstruction, the upper extent of the lesion is not visualized. While the upper extent is of less importance to the neurosurgeon, who is able to extend his incision as required to decompress the cord, it is of great concern to the radiation therapist who has to devise the appropriate treatment field. If radiation therapy is to be used as the first treatment modality, introduction of contrast material through a cervical or cisternal puncture is recommended to establish the upper limit of the obstruction. The optimal treatment for a spinal cord compression depends on the clinical presentation. Radiation therapy can be instituted in patients with early or slowly progressive symptoms, or in patients with involvement below the conus medullaris, with laminectomy reserved for patients who fail to improve. Surgery is recommended for patients with severe or rapidly progressive symptoms, after which radiation is used, since surgery rarely results in complete removal of the tumor. When radiation therapy is chosen for the initial treatment, administration of high-dose corticosteroids (Decadron, 4 mg qid or greater) is recommended prior to the first treatment, to prevent possible progression of symptoms secondary to radiation-induced edema. Response to treatment is highly dependent on the degree, duration, and rapidity of symptoms. Of patients diagnosed prior to the development of motor loss, approximately 60 percent remain ambulatory. In contrast, only a third of paretic patients become ambulatory, and paraplegic patients only rarely return to ambulation. These figures underscore the importance of early diagnosis and treatment of this complication.

Treatment of Intracranial Metastases

Intracranial metastases are a frequent occurrence in patients with metastatic carcinoma of the breast. Less commonly, intracranial metastases occur as the first manifestation of metastatic disease. Patients are seen in a variety of clinical settings, depending on the site of intracranial involvement. Headache, nausea, vomiting, and visual disturbances, all suggesting increased intracranial pressure, are frequently present. Physical examination correspondingly reflects the site of involvement as well as varying degrees of papilledema. The diagnosis is confirmed by a conventional brain scan, CT brain scan, or, less commonly, arteriography. In the rare situation in which a single lesion is detected and the patient has no other metastatic disease, a craniotomy is sometimes warranted to establish the diagnosis. In most situations, however, the diagnosis is made on clinical grounds, and patients are spared craniotomy. The optimal treatment is whole brain radiation since small, undetectable lesions are invariably present in other parts of the brain. Patients usually receive 300 rads per day to a total of 3000 rads over $2\frac{1}{2}$ weeks. On occasion areas of gross disease receive higher doses through a smaller field. As with spinal cord compression, high-dose corticosteroids are given prior to the first treatment.

Treatment of Superior Mediastinal Compression

Because of the anatomic constraints in the superior mediastinum, malignant lymphadenopathy occurring in this region can result in compression of vital structures such as the superior vena cava, trachea, or esophagus. Patients with compression of the superior vena cava present with edema of the head and neck, while patients with compression of the trachea or esophagus present with dyspnea or dysphagia. Further evaluation, such as brachial venography or mediastinoscopy, is discouraged because of the significant risk of thrombosis and hemorrhage. This clinical condition is progressive and fatal if untreated. The diagnosis is made solely on clinical grounds, and treatment should be instituted promptly. If superior vena caval compression is detected at an early stage, mediastinal radiation is effective at reversing symptoms. In advanced cases, especially when thrombosis has developed, radiation is less effective.

Miscellaneous

Brachial Plexus

Involvement of the brachial plexus can occur in patients with metastases to the axillary apex or supraclavicular lymph nodes. Patients are initially seen with distal paresthesias and show progressive motor loss and pain. Radiation treatment is delivered by means of opposing anterior and posterior fields extending superiorly to the midneck. In patients who have not received previous cervical spine radiation, this region is included in the treatment field. If the cervical spine has been previously irradiated, the fields are obliquely angled in order to cover the supraclavicular region and axillary apex without treating the cervical spinal cord. The recommended dose is 4000 to 5000 rads over 4 to 5 weeks. Additional treatment by means of a smaller field is sometimes attempted in patients who have not shown a significant improvement following administration of 5000 rads. In a response similar to that of other complications, brachial plexus symptoms can be reversed if treated at an early stage. Treatment can be ineffective at relieving symptoms in more advanced cases with extensive tumor destruction of the brachial plexus.

Choroid, Retina, and Retroorbital Areas

Metastases from carcinoma of the breast have a predilection for the choroid, retina, and retroorbital areas. Patients with choroidal or retinal involvement are first seen with decreasing vision, and fundoscopic examination will confirm the diagnosis. Radiation treatment is delivered by means of a direct anterior field with the patient's eyes open during treatment. Since radiation-induced cataract formation takes many years to occur and survival in this group of patients is so limited, radiation to the cornea has not been a significant problem. Patients commonly receive 3000 to 4000 rads over $2^1/_2$ to 4 weeks. Retroorbital involvement may be first seen with proptosis, with or without decreasing vision. The diagnosis is confirmed by retroorbital ultrasonography or by a CT scan of the retroorbital region. Since involvement is frequently bilateral, treatment is delivered by means of opposed lateral fields to both retroorbital spaces. The recommended dose is 3000 rads over $2^1/_2$ weeks.

Liver

Liver involvement due to metastatic carcinoma of the breast may be so massive as to result in significant right upper quadrant pain. This pain is believed to result from parenchymal enlargement and stretching of the liver capsule. In our experience, this pain is effectively treated by radiation. Patients receive 300 rads per day, 4 days per week, for 2 weeks. After six treatments, the field is narrowed to avoid further radiation to the left kidney. When radiation treatment is restricted to the liver itself with minimal bowel exposure, significant nausea and vomiting are not encountered.

References

1. Bonadonna, G., Valagussa, P., Rossi, A., et al. Are surgical adjuvant trials altering the course of breast cancer? *Semin. Oncol.* 5:450, 1978.
2. Bruckman, J. E., Harris, J. R., Levene, M. B., et al. Results of treating stage III carcinoma of the breast by primary radiation therapy. *Cancer* 43:985, 1979.
3. Chu, F. C. H., Lin, F. J., Kim, J. H., et al. Locally recurrent carcinoma of the breast. *Cancer* 37:2677, 1976.
4. Fisher, B., Slack, N. H., and Cavanaugh, P. J. Post-operative radiotherapy in the treatment of breast cancer: Results of the NSABP clinical trial. *Ann. Surg.* 172:711, 1970.
5. Fletcher, G. H., *Textbook of Radiotherapy.* Philadelphia: Lea & Febiger, 1973.
6. Haagensen, C. D., Miller, E., Handley, R. S., et al. Treatment of early breast cancer: A cooperative international study. *Ann. Surg.* 170:875, 1969.
7. Haagensen, C. D., and Stout, A. P. Carcinoma of the breast: Criteria of operability. *Ann. Surg.* 118:859, 1943.
8. Harris, J. R., Levene, M. B., and Hellman, S. The role of radiation therapy in the primary treatment of carcinoma of the breast. *Semin. Oncol.* 5:403, 1978.

9. Harris, J. R., Levene, M. B., and Hellman, S. Results of treating stage I and II carcinoma of the breast with primary radiation therapy. *Cancer Treat. Rep.* 62:985, 1978.

10. Harris, J. R., Levene, M. B., Svensson, G., et al. Analysis of cosmetic results following primary radiation therapy for stages I and II carcinoma of the breast. *Int. J. Radiat. Oncol. Biol. Phys.* 5:257, 1979.

11. Mustakallio, S. Conservative treatment of breast cancer—Review of 25 years follow up. *Clin. Radiol.* 23:110, 1972.

12. Peters, M. V. Cutting the "Gordian knot" in early breast cancer. *Ann. R. Coll. Phys. Surg. Can.* 8:186, 1975.

13. Pierquin, B., Baillet, F., and Wilson, J. F. Radiation therapy in the management of primary breast cancer. *A.J.R.* 127:645, 1976.

14. Piro, A. J., and Hellman, S. Effect of primary treatment modality on the metastatic pattern of mammary carcinoma. *Cancer Treat. Rep.* 62:1275, 1978.

15. Spitalier, J., Brandone, H., Ayme, Y., et al. Cesiumtherapy of breast cancer. A five-year report of 400 consecutive patients. *Int. J. Radiat. Oncol. Biol. Phys.* 2:231, 1977.

16. Spratt, J. S., and Donegan, W. L. *Cancer of the Breast.* St. Louis: C. V. Mosby, 1967.

17. Valagussa, P., Bonadonna, G., and Veronesi, V. Patterns of relapse and survival following radical mastectomy. *Cancer* 41:1170, 1978.

18. Weichselbaum, R. R., Marck, A., and Hellman, S. The role of post-operative irradiation in carcinoma of the breast. *Cancer* 37:2682, 1976.

19. Zimmerman, K. W., Montague, E. D., and Fletcher, G. H. Frequency, anatomical distribution and management of local recurrences after definitive therapy for breast cancer. *Cancer* 19:67, 1966.

George P. Canellos
I. Craig Henderson

10. Medical Management of Advanced Breast Cancer

Management of Disseminated Disease— Prognostic Factors that Predict Relapse

Only about 50 percent of the patients with what appears to be localized primary breast cancer will be alive and free of disease 10 years after their initial diagnosis [54]. Further, the precise type and combination of surgery and radiation therapy does not appear to affect these survival figures.

The progressive relapse rate over more than 20 years probably reflects the heterogeneity of the growth rate of micrometastasis. Analysis of clinical and pathologic data has permitted identification of groups of patients in whom the risks of relapse may be roughly predicted. Patients with tumors less than 2 cm in diameter without histologic axillary lymph node involvement have an excellent 10-year survival rate, approaching 90 percent in some series. Unfortunately, this group of patients is small (about 10 percent). In the vast majority of patients, the tumors are 2 to 5 cm in diameter, and about half of these patients have axillary node involvement as well. The risk of subsequent recurrence of disease has been correlated with a number of clinical and pathologic factors; these include: (1) tumor size, (2) presence of tumor in the axillary lymph nodes, (3) the histologic grade of differentiation, (4) the presence of blood vessel invasion, (5) the presence of sinus histiocytosis in the axillary lymph nodes, (6) lymphoid cell infiltration of the tumor, (7) perinodal infiltration of the tumor in the axilla, and (8) the presence of the estrogen receptor protein. Only the first two of these, however, are universally accepted as being useful in the clinical management of breast cancer.

Larger primary tumors are associated with a higher incidence and larger number of involved axillary nodes, a shorter disease-free interval, and a greater likelihood of local recurrence [11, 54]. The incidence of axillary node involvement in lesions less than 2 cm in diameter (T1*) is about 40 percent and increases to about 55 percent in patients with lesions of more than 2 cm. Involvement of the axillary nodes by tumor increases the risk of relapse independent of tumor size [47]. Although some investigators believe that a single positive node may not increase the risk of relapse, several studies do not support this hypothesis. In premenopausal women, a single involved node confers a likelihood of relapse almost equal to the presence of two or three positive nodes, and the risk of relapse increases markedly when four or more nodes contain tumor [9, 52]. Extranodal extension of tumor from the axillary nodes may also be a poor prognostic sign, but this is usually seen in patients with many involved nodes [20].

The histopathologic features of the primary tumor can influence prognosis. In some series, patients with anaplastic tumors did poorly in contrast to those with well-differentiated lesions. The demonstration of sinus histiocytosis in axillary nodes was shown to be correlated with perivenous lymphoid infiltration in the primary tumor, and it is possible that both of these characteristics confer a more favorable prognosis, perhaps representing a cellular hypersensitivity response to the patient's tumor [8].

The endocrine status of the patient and the tumor may predict relapse within a defined period. The Milan data [9] suggests that the rate of relapse occurs earlier among premenopausal women. Patients with tumors lacking the estrogen receptor protein (ERP) have also been found to relapse at a faster rate than those with ERP positive tumors [37]. Since tumors arising in premenopausal women are likely to be ERP negative, there is probably an association between these two observations. Thymidine-labeling studies suggest that greater proliferative activity occurs when the estrogen receptor is absent [38]. Tumors with an ERP therefore may have a slower rate of proliferation, even if dissemination has occurred. The pattern of relapse and distribution to metastatic sites does not differ between axillary node–positive and node–negative patients. Local-regional relapse (25 percent of all cases) is more likely in node-positive patients with large primary tumors. In such node-positive patients, osseous metastases occur in a median time of 2.4 years,

*See Chapter 2 for TNM staging criteria from which this is taken.

but multiple visceral metastases will occur earlier, at about 1.1 years. Most local recurrences will occur within 3 years, and the vast majority of this group of node-positive patients will also show distant metastases within the next 2 years [54]. Axillary node–negative patients will demonstrate fewer local recurrences, but distant metastases will be equally distributed between bone and multiple visceral sites.

Endocrine Therapy for Metastatic Disease
Hormonal Ablation
Determination of the presence of the estrogen receptor protein on tumor cells has allowed for selection of patients likely to respond to hormonal treatment. The additional presence of a progesterone receptor may increase the likelihood of a hormonal response [37]. The earliest form of hormonal therapy was castration in premenopausal women. The general experience with this operation indicated that 30 to 40 percent of the patients sustained a response of varying quality that usually lasted less than 12 months.

The clinical pattern of disease likely to respond to castration includes a long disease-free interval followed by metastases to bone, lymph nodes, and soft tissue. Patients with disease in the liver, brain, and peritoneum are less likely to benefit. Patients with single metastatic sites responded more often than those with multiple sites [44]. Responders lived longer than nonresponders, since subsequent hormonal manipulations were more likely to be successful [29]. The single most important subjective complaint that may dramatically improve is bone pain. Use of the estrogen receptor assay will predict response in about 60 percent of patients [33].

Adrenalectomy has been employed since 1952 as a secondary endocrine ablative procedure in premenopausal women and as a primary node in selected postmenopausal women [46, 48]. Some prefer to combine oophorectomy and adrenalectomy in a single procedure in their patients. A review of the larger series concludes that without the benefit of estrogen receptor assay, the likelihood of response to adrenalectomy is greater in patients under 50 years of age, those with a previous oophorectomy response, those with a disease-free interval longer than 2 years, and those with a single metastatic site. Those with metastases to the liver and central nervous system (CNS) have a distinctly lower response rate [46, 48]. Overall, about one third of patients respond to the procedure, but the regression rate is higher in estrogen receptor positive patients [33]. The median survival of responders is 26 months, while less than 10 months in nonresponders.

It is now possible to ablate adrenal steroid production medically. Aminoglutethimide inhibits the adrenal conversion of cholesterol to pregnenolone [45]; a dose of 250 mg four times a day will effectively inhibit adrenal steroid production, and simultaneous glucocorticoid administration will inhibit adrenocorticotropic hormone (ACTH) elaboration. A combination of agents is capable of inducing regressions in metastatic breast cancer in 30 to 40 percent of patients [45, 51]. If this combination is used for a finite period of time (3 months), response to it can accurately predict future response to adrenalectomy [42]. More recently, cortisone, hydrocortisone, or both, have replaced dexamethasone as the replacement glucocorticoid of choice, since it was found that aminoglutethimide accelerated the metabolism of the latter [45]. Medical adrenalectomy has rapidly replaced the surgical approach, especially in postmenopausal patients. The risk of subjecting a patient to the morbidity of a major ablative procedure must be balanced against the benefits and availability of other modes of therapy. It is important to emphasize that although responders to ablation survive longer than nonresponders, a randomized comparison of postmenopausal women showed no survival advantage when surgical adrenalectomy was compared with medical ablation and additive hormones [55]. "Prophylactic" or adjuvant oophorectomy has not been shown to increase survival [26].

Hypophysectomy is not commonly used to effect hormonal ablation because of the availability of other treatment modalities. It appears to be as effective as adrenalectomy, although replacement therapy for hypophysectomy can become complicated and require the supervision of an endocrinologist. The response rate is again 30 to 40 percent and is greater than this in receptor positive patients. Of interest is the fact that measurements of pituitary-derived peptide hormones show a decrease, but rarely a total absence, following transphenoid hypophysectomy. There does not appear to be a correlation between response and completeness of ablation [7, 32].

Hormonal Agents

The use of hormonal agents to treat breast cancer has undergone a rapid metamorphosis since the introduction of orally effective estrogen antagonists. In the past, only androgens and estrogens of varying potency were available. The primary role of these hormones was in the postmenopausal patient with osseous or soft tissue metastases. The response rate to extrinsic hormones increases as a function of time from menopause and correlates with the presence of the ERP. The use of androgens is rapidly declining, their effectiveness limited by the masculinizing side effects as well as disturbing abnormalities in liver function, increased libido in elderly women, and secondary polycythemia [32]. The most commonly used androgen is fluoxymesterone (Halotestin) in a dose range of 10 mg taken twice a day.

The precise mechanism of action is unknown, but there is general agreement that estrogens probably provide the more effective of the two therapies. The principal limitation is gastrointestinal intolerance, but the other toxic side effects include fluid retention, breast engorgement, softening of the skin, and diarrhea. Rarely a serious hypercalcemia crisis can be induced by the initiation of estrogen therapy [27]. The most commonly used agent is diethylstilbestrol, 5 mg taken three times a day. In patients with disseminated disease who are on estrogen therapy and develop further progression, sudden cessation of estrogen may produce regression. This withdrawal response can occur in up to 30 percent of patients [5]. Progestational agents such as medroxyprogesterone acetate have been used in high doses with varying success [31]. There have been uncontrolled trials that claim that the addition of progestational agents to estrogens can achieve a higher response rate [16]. These and other combinations of hormonal agents have not been shown to be superior to single agent therapy [16, 28].

Antiestrogens

The antiestrogenic compounds in clinical use include nafoxidine and tamoxifen citrate. The former, although effective, has not achieved wide acceptance because of its associated toxicity, including partial hair loss, skin dryness, icthyosis, and acquired photosensitivity [34]. These compounds were demonstrated in vitro to inhibit the uptake of estradiol in experimental and human tumors. They have the capacity to bind to the estrogen receptor and form a complex that in turn binds to nuclear chromatin. These compounds bear a structural resemblance to potent estrogens such as stilbestrol, and mild estrogenic effects have been noted when they are used in high doses [33]. These antiestrogenic compounds have their greatest effect in patients with estrogen receptor positive tumors [40].

Tamoxifen citrate is quickly becoming the most widely used oral antihormonal agent. It has been used primarily in treating postmenopausal women. When used in a dosage range of 10 to 20 mg taken twice daily, an objective response rate of approximately 30 to 40 percent has been noted [21]. The mean duration of response varies widely from several months to over 2 years. Most series include patients who were previously treated with other hormones, and prior response to other endocrine therapies appears to predict response to tamoxifen citrate. Failure to respond to estrogens or androgens does not preclude a response to tamoxifen citrate [21]. Sites of involvement responding to this agent include soft tissue, bone, skin, and lung.

Whether there is value in using this agent in patients who have previously responded to adrenalectomy or hypophysectomy is unknown [36]. Information concerning the converse approach is sparse but important, since tamoxifen citrate may be of value in predicting subsequent response to adrenalectomy or hypophysectomy. There is a report that 1 of 5 patients responded to hypophysectomy after failing to respond to tamoxifen citrate [36]. The side effects of this agent are generally quite mild and include nausea, hot flashes, vaginal discharge, hypercalcemia, and transient thrombocytopenia. It is currently being added to chemotherapy regimens for advanced disease but does not appear to have enhanced the activity of cytotoxic drugs [23].

Cytotoxic Chemotherapy

Disseminated breast cancer is one of the malignancies most responsive to cytotoxic cancer chemotherapeutic agents. Responses have been reported for a variety of agents with differing biochemical mechanisms of action. They include the alkylating agents cyclophosphamide, chlorambucil, phenylalanine mustard, and thiotepa; the antimetabolites 5-fluorouracil (5-FU) and methotrexate; and Adriamycin. The vinca alkaloids have a low order of activity but have been included in some combination chemotherapy programs. All of these drugs have been used as single agents in patients previously treated with radiation and hormonal agents; in that setting, the response rate varies from 20 to 25 percent, depending on the agent, patient selectivity, and the extent of measurable disease. Almost all of the responses have been partial responses, and, in most instances, cross-resistance amongst these agents has not been seen. The fact that a variety of agents was useful justified their inclusion in combined drug programs for advanced breast cancer.

The most effective combination chemotherapy programs include at least cyclophosphamide and 5-fluorouracil. Initially, four cytotoxic drugs were combined with prednisone in the so-called Cooper regimen, which consisted of cyclophosphamide, methotrexate, 5-fluorouracil, vincristine, and prednisone. Subsequent reports have included investigations of varying combinations of agents given in different doses and schedules, with approximately the same results for each. In patients not previously treated with cytotoxic agents, any combination chemotherapy program composed of these agents is capable of inducing a response in approximately 50 to 70 percent. This would appear to produce better results than single drug chemotherapy. In one randomized trial the combination of three drugs—cyclophosphamide, methotrexate, and 5-fluorouracil (CMF)—was shown to be superior to a single alkylating agent, L-phenylalanine mustard (L-PAM) [14]. However, the survival rates between two randomized groups did not differ significantly, except in those patients who had liver metastases or who were otherwise nonambulatory.

Results of administration of single agents delivered sequentially versus the same agents delivered in combinations have been studied, but neither regimen demonstrated superiority in overall survival at 2 years [6, 50]. In one trial, however, the median survival in the combination chemotherapy groups appeared to be superior to that in the group in which the single agent was given sequentially. In addition, the overall response rate was higher [50]. Combination chemotherapy programs, too, have achieved complete responses in up to 30 percent of patients, which is rare with single agents. Although it is difficult to show a difference in survival between complete and partial responders, most trials demonstrate that both have a survival superior to that of nonresponders. Although a variety of dosages and schedules is available, it is difficult to identify a combination program that is clearly superior to all others [15].

Ideally, a combination chemotherapy program should be administered on an outpatient basis, have tolerable toxicity, and be given in a schedule that allows for maximum effectiveness of the agents. The CMF program is composed of cyclophosphamide given in a daily oral dose of 100 mg/M^2 for 14 days out of a 28-day cycle; methotrexate 60 mg/M^2 given intravenously on days 1 and 8 of a 28-day cycle; and 5-fluorouracil 600 mg/M^2 given intravenously on days 1 and 8 of the 28-day cycle. The various combinations employing at least these three drugs or variations composed of cyclophosphamide, 5-fluorouracil, and prednisone indicate that responses are usually seen within the first two cycles of chemotherapy [15]. The median duration of response varies from 8 to 16 months, and most patients require intermittent chemotherapy because of the paucity of complete remissions. The addition of vincristine to these programs has not appeared to increase the response rate, and the neurotoxicity associated with it has discouraged its inclusion in most programs [1].

The evaluation of Adriamycin in prospective randomized trials indicates that it is probably the most active single agent in the treatment of breast cancer. The response rate varies from 33 to 52 percent when 60 to 75 mg/M^2 is given every 3 weeks, with the responses lasting from 5 to 8 months [24]. The combination chemotherapy programs that include Adriamycin, cyclophosphamide, and 5-fluorouracil demonstrate a higher average response rate than Adriamycin alone, but the duration of response is not improved [24, 25, 53]. Trials comparing combinations composed of varied mixtures of cyclophosphamide, methotrexate, 5-FU, Adriamycin, prednisone, and vincristine have not clearly demonstrated that one of these combinations is superior in overall response and survival [1, 10, 13, 41, 49]. The toxic effects of all of these combination programs include myelosuppression, mucositis, neurotoxicity, and rarely cardiomyopathy associated with Adriamycin. The degrees of myelosuppression will vary with the prior treatment status of the patient, her age, and whether radiation therapy has been previously administered to the spine and pelvis.

In patients with rapidly progressive disease involving the liver, lung, and other visceral organs, prompt therapy is necessary. When a response might be life-saving and is required in a short period of time, it is clear that combination chemotherapy should be considered in preference to single agents.

The demonstrated superiority of combination chemotherapy in terms of response rate over single agents suggests that they produce a greater initial destruction of tumor cells. Thus, it appears advisable to employ regimens offering the maximum antitumor response as adjuvants to primary therapy, whether it be surgery or radiation.

There is little clinical information that can predict a response to cytotoxic chemotherapy. It is difficult to assess the responsiveness of bone lesions to chemotherapy, but with the advent of combination chemotherapy, healing has been reported in those patients who achieved an excellent systemic response. There is controversy as to whether the estrogen receptor protein can predict a response to chemotherapy. Series defending both the predictability or lack of predictability of the estrogen receptor have been reported [4, 30]. If, however, one uses response to hormonal treatment alone as a basis of predictability, it appears not to predict for a subsequent response to cytotoxic agents [22]. The presence or absence of an estrogen receptor is not relevant to a decision to use cytotoxic chemotherapy if hormone therapy is not otherwise indicated or has been tried unsuccessfully. An interesting trial from Britain randomized patients between combination chemotherapy and hormonal therapy as a first treatment without regard for estrogen receptor content. It is noteworthy that the overall survival between the two groups did not differ, although cytotoxic treatment gave a higher response rate. In premenopausal patients, however, the cytotoxically treated group appeared to do considerably better than those patients who had an ovarian ablation [43]. Prior treatment with cytotoxic agents does not interfere with hormonal response [43].

It has been difficult to establish whether the addition of hormonal manipulation to cytotoxic chemotherapy increases the response rate or its duration. A randomized trial in premeno-

pausal women in which oophorectomy plus combination chemotherapy was compared with combination chemotherapy alone
suggests an advantage for the combined treatment [12]. Similarly, in premenopausal women, the addition of chemotherapy
to oophorectomy as an early adjunct to that procedure improves
the response rate and the progression-free duration when compared with combination chemotherapy given only at the time
of progression following oophorectomy [2]. The progression-
free intervals between the two treatment groups were 53 and
17 weeks, respectively. In postmenopausal women, it is difficult
to demonstrate any advantage to adding hormonal treatments
such as diethylstilbestrol or progesterone to cytotoxic agents
[12]. One uncontrolled trial appeared to demonstrate a superiority compared to other series when combination chemotherapy was added to hormonal procedures, with 51 percent
complete responders who survived a median duration of 27
months [35]. It is clear that the addition of cytotoxic chemotherapy to hormonal management may increase the duration of
control of disease. However, to date there is no evidence that
supports the fact that the combined modalities result in a better
long-term disease-free survival.

Adjuvant Treatment

The use of adjuvant therapy is based on experimental data that
demonstrate a greater likelihood for eradication of residual disease when it exists only as micrometastases. The value of adjuvant therapy can only be appreciated in randomized trials
composed of adequate numbers of patients properly stratified
who are compared with patients in a similar control group that
is not treated. It was such a randomized trial that demonstrated
that postoperative radiation therapy did not contribute to the
survival of patients but only decreased the incidence of local
recurrence [18]. Local recurrences can be effectively treated by
radiation therapy, but they are rarely the only sites of recurrence.

Early adjuvant chemotherapy series were begun in the late
1950s when small doses of alkylating agents were given at the
time of surgery. In one study, adjuvant therapy consisted of
thiotepa, 0.4 mg/kg, given on the day of surgery, followed in
two successive days by doses of 0.2 mg/kg as the sole systemic

treatment [19]. This study indicated a marginal advantage in overall survival for premenopausal women with four or more positive nodes who were followed to 10 years. A Scandinavian study [39] employed a total dose of 30 mg/kg of cyclophosphamide spread over 6 days at the time of surgery. This trial has demonstrated a statistically significant difference in the recurrence rate between the treated and controlled group, but the differences are no greater than 10 percent. It is apparent that small amounts of chemotherapy given soon after surgery require prolonged periods of follow-up with large numbers of patients to demonstrate a small advantage.

The two major controlled adjuvant trials are those of Fisher [17] and Bonadonna [9]. The Fisher trial employed L-phenyl-alanine mustard (L-PAM) at 0.15 mg/kg per day for 5 consecutive days every 6 weeks for 2 years. When this treatment was begun no later than 4 weeks after surgery and compared with placebo treatment, an advantage in disease-free survival was noted in patients less than 49 years of age who had one to three positive nodes at the time of mastectomy. In a more recent trial [9], the addition of 5-FU at 300 mg/M^2 per day given intravenously for 5 consecutive days every 6 weeks was compared in a randomized fashion to L-PAM. It is too early to ascertain the impact of the second drug, however. A Mayo Clinic trial comparing L-PAM with cyclophosphamide, 5-FU and prednisone as adjuvants to primary therapy is showing an advantage for the combined drug approach in premenopausal women [3], but the follow-up period barely exceeds 2 years. The National Cancer Institute of Milan embarked on a prospective randomized trial in which 12 months on the CMF program was compared with no treatment in a group of patients who had received radical mastectomies [9]. The trial began in June of 1973 and was terminated in September of 1975 after an accrual of 386 patients. At the present time there remains a statistically significant difference between the treated and control groups. An approximately 20 percent difference at 5 years in relapse-free survival is highly significant. The differences are more striking in the premenopausal group; only 25 percent of the premenopausal patients treated with CMF relapsed in 4 years, compared with 59 percent of the control group. These differences apply to all the subgroups rated according to the number of positive axillary nodes. There also appears to be a statistically significant difference in survival, as well as disease-free survival, at 4 years.

Carefully administered chemotherapy in this age group should result in similar benefit. It is clear that cytotoxic agents are effective in postmenopausal patients with disseminated disease. It may be only a matter of further follow-up before a statistical advantage will be noted. The optimal duration of adjuvant chemotherapy is unknown. There appeared to be no difference in results of trials of 6 months and 12 months of CMF after approximately 2 years of follow-up [9]. Clearly, better adjuvant therapy is required. Of interest is the fact that despite the omission of radiation therapy in the Milan trial, the local-regional relapse rate appears to be no greater than that seen with adjuvant radiation therapy (5 to 8 percent).

Adjuvant chemotherapy affects the menstrual cycle of premenopausal women, resulting in amenorrhea in approximately 80 percent of patients; this is irreversible in about 20 percent, especially in women less than 40 years of age. The Milan data indicates a correlation, although not a statistically significant one, between amenorrhea and disease-free survival at 4 years; this suggests that better results are seen in patients becoming amenorrheic. When the Milan data are compared with results of adjuvant castration studies, chemotherapy treatment appears to be superior.

The results of these trials suggest that premenopausal women with positive axillary nodes or stage III disease being controlled by local surgery and radiation therapy should receive chemotherapy as an adjuvant to primary treatment.

References

1. Ahmann, D. L., Bisel, H. F., Eagan, R. T., et al. Controlled evaluation of Adriamycin (NSC-123127) in patients with disseminated breast cancer. *Cancer Chemother. Rep.* 58:877, 1974.
2. Ahmann, D. L., O'Connell, M. J., Hahn, R. G., et al. An evaluation of early or delayed adjuvant chemotherapy in premenopausal patients with advanced breast cancer undergoing oophorectomy. *N. Engl. J. Med.* 297:356, 1977.
3. Ahmann, D. L., Scanlon, P. W., Bisel, H. F., et al. Repeated adjuvant chemotherapy with phenylalanine mustard or 5-fluorouracil, cyclophosphamide, and prednisone with or without radiation, after mastectomy for breast cancer. *Lancet* 1:893, 1978.
4. Allegra, J. C., Lippman, M. E., Thompson, E. B., and Simon, R.

An association between steroid hormone receptors and response to cytotoxic chemotherapy in patients with metastatic breast cancer. *Cancer Res.* 38:4299, 1978.

5. Baker, L. H., and Vaitkevicius, V. K. Reevaluation of rebound regression in disseminated carcinoma of the breast. *Cancer* 29:1268, 1972.

6. Baker, L. H., Vaughn, C. B., Al-Sarraf, M., et al. Evaluation of combination vs. sequential cytotoxic chemotherapy in the treatment of advanced breast cancer. *Cancer* 33:513, 1974.

7. Bates, T., Rubens, R. D., Bulbrook, R. D., et al. Comparison of pituitary function and clinical response after transphenoidal and transfrontal hypophysectomy for advanced breast cancer. *Eur. J. Cancer* 12:775, 1976.

8. Black, M. M., Barclay, T. H., and Hankev, B. F. Prognosis in breast cancer utilizing histologic characteristics of the primary tumor. *Cancer* 36:2048, 1975.

9. Bonadonna, G., Valagussa, P., Rossi, A., et al. Are surgical adjuvant trials altering the course of breast cancer? *Sem. Oncol.* 5:450, 1978.

10. Brambilla, C., DeLena, M., Rossi, A., et al. Response and survival in advanced breast cancer after two non-cross-resistant combinations. *Br. Med. J.* 1:801, 1976.

11. Breast Cancer Study Group. Identification of breast cancer patients with high risk of early recurrence after radical mastectomy. *Cancer* 42:2809, 1978.

12. Brunner, K. W., Sonntag, R. W., Alberto, P., et al. Combined chemo- and hormonal therapy in advanced breast cancer. *Cancer* 39:2923, 1977.

13. Bull, J. M., Tormey, D. C., Li, S., et al. A randomized comparative trial of adriamycin versus methotrexate in combination drug therapy. *Cancer* 41:1649, 1978.

14. Canellos, G. P., Pocock, S. J., Taylor, S. G., et al. Combination chemotherapy for metastatic breast carcinoma. *Cancer* 38:1882, 1976.

15. Carter, S. K. Integration of chemotherapy into combined modality treatment of solid tumors. *Cancer Treat. Rev.* 3:141, 1976.

16. Crowley, L. G., and MacDonald, I. Delalutin and estrogens for the treatment of advanced mammary carcinoma of the postmenopausal woman. *Cancer* 18:436, 1965.

17. Fisher, B., Glass, A., Redmond, C., et al. L-phenylalanine mustard (L-PAM) in the management of primary breast cancer. *Cancer* 39:2883, 1977.

18. Fisher, B., Slack, N. H., Cavanaugh, P. J., et al. Post-operative radiotherapy in the treatment of breast cancer: Results of the NSABP clinical trial. *Ann. Surg.* 172:711, 1970.

19. Fisher, B., Slack, N., Katrych, D., and Wolmark, N. Ten year follow-up results of patients with carcinoma of the breast in a cooperative clinical trial evaluating surgical adjuvant chemotherapy. *Surg. Gynecol. Obstet.* 140:528, 1975.

20. Fisher, E. R., Gregorio, R. M., Redmond, C., et al. Pathologic findings from the national surgical adjuvant breast project. *Am. J. Clin. Pathol.* 65:439, 1976.
21. Heel, R. C., Brogden, R. N., Speight, T. M., and Avery, G. S. Tamoxifen: A review of its pharmacological properties and therapeutic use in the treatment of breast cancer. *Drugs* 16:1, 1978.
22. Henderson, M. D., Buroker, T. R., Samson, M. K., et al. Response of patients with carcinoma of the breast to hormonal therapy and combination chemotherapy. *Surg. Gynecol. Obstet.* 141:232, 1975.
23. Heuson, J. Current overview of EORTC clinical trials with Tamoxifen. *Cancer Treat. Rep.* 60:1463, 1976.
24. Hoogstraten, B., George, S. L., Samal, B., et al. Combination chemotherapy and adriamycin in patients with advanced breast cancer. *Cancer* 38:13, 1976.
25. Kennealey, G. T., Boston, B., Mitchell, M. S., et al. Combination chemotherapy for advanced breast cancer. *Cancer* 42:27, 1978.
26. Kennedy, B. J. Hormone therapy for advanced breast cancer. *Cancer* 18:1551, 1965.
27. Kennedy, B. J. Hormonal therapies in breast cancer. *Sem. Oncol.* 1:119, 1974.
28. Kennedy, B. J., and Brown, J. H. Combined estrogenic and androgenic hormone therapy in advanced breast cancer. *Cancer* 18:431, 1965.
29. Kennedy, B. J., and Fortuny, I. E. Therapeutic castration in the treatment of advanced breast cancer. *Cancer* 17:1197, 1964.
30. Kiang, D. T., Frenning, D. H., Goldman, A. I., et al. Estrogen receptors and responses to chemotherapy and hormonal therapy in advanced breast cancer. *N. Engl. J. Med.* 299:1330, 1978.
31. Klaassen, D. J., Rapp, E. F., and Hirte, W. E. Response to medroxyprogesterone acetate (NSC026383) as secondary hormone therapy for metastatic breast cancer in postmenopausal women. *Cancer Treat. Rep.* 60:251, 1976.
32. LaRossa, J. T., Strong, M. S., and Melby, J. C. Endocrinologically incomplete transethmoidal trans-sphenoidal hypophysectomy with relief of bone pain in breast cancer. *N. Engl. J. Med.* 298:1332, 1978.
33. Legha, S. S., Davis, H. L., and Muggia, F. M. Hormonal therapy breast cancer: New approaches and concepts. *Ann. Intern. Med.* 88:69, 1978.
34. Legha, S. S., Slavik, M., and Carter, S. K. Nafoxidine—an antiestrogen for the treatment of breast cancer. *Cancer* 38:1535, 1976.
35. Mannes, P., Derriks, R., Moens, R., et al. Multidisciplinary curative treatment for disseminated carcinoma of the breast. *Cancer Treat. Rep.* 60:85, 1976.
36. Manni, A., Trujillo, J., Marshall, J. S., and Pearson, O. H. Antiestrogen-induced remission in stage IV breast cancer. *Cancer Treat. Rep.* 60:1445, 1976.

37. McGuire, W. L. Hormone receptors: Their role in predicting prognosis and response to endocrine therapy. *Sem. Oncol.* 5:428, 1978.
38. Meyer, J. S., Rao, B. R., Stevens, S. C., and White, W. L. Low incidence of estrogen receptor in breast carcinomas with rapid rates of cellular replication. *Cancer* 40:2290, 1977.
39. Meyer, R., Kjellgren, K., Malmio, K., et al. Surgical adjuvant chemotherapy. *Cancer* 41:2088, 1978.
40. Moseson, D. L., Sasaki, G. H., and Kraybill, W. G., et al. The use of antiestrogens Tamoxifen and nafoxidine in the treatment of human breast cancer in correlation with estrogen receptor values. *Cancer* 41:797, 1978.
41. Nemoto, T., Rosner, D., Diaz, R., et al. Combination chemotherapy for metastatic breast cancer. *Cancer* 41:2073, 1978.
42. Newsome, H. H., Brown, P. W., Terz, J. J., and Lawrence, W., Jr. Medical and surgical adrenalectomy in patients with advanced breast carcinoma. *Cancer* 39:542, 1977.
43. Priestman, T., Baum, M., Jones, V., and Forbes, J. Treatment and survival in advanced breast cancer. *Br. Med. J.* 2:1673, 1978.
44. Puga, F. J., Welch, J. S., and Bisel, H. F. Therapeutic oophorectomy in disseminated carcinoma of the breast. *Arch. Surg.* 111:877, 1976.
45. Santen, R. J., Samojlik, E., Lipton, A., et al. Kinetic hormonal and clinical studies with aminoglutethimide in breast cancer. *Cancer* 39:2948, 1977.
46. Schmidt, M., Nemoto, T., Dao, T., and Bross, I. D. J. Prognostic factors affecting adrenalectomy in patients with metastatic cancer of the breast. *Cancer* 27:1106, 1971.
47. Schottenfeld, D., Nash, A. G., Robbins, G. F., and Beattie, E. J., Jr. Ten-year survival of the treatment of primary operable breast carcinoma. *Cancer* 38:1001, 1976.
48. Silverstein, M. J., Byron, R. L., Jr., Yonemoto, R. H., et al. Bilateral adrenalectomy for advanced breast cancer: A 21-year experience. *Surgery* 77:825, 1977.
49. Smalley, R. V., Carpenter, J., Bartolucci, A., et al. A comparison of cyclophosphamide, adriamycin, 5-fluorouracil (CAF) and cyclophosphamide, vincristine, and prednisone (CMFVP) in patients with metastatic breast cancer. *Cancer* 40:625, 1977.
50. Smalley, R. V., Murphy, S., Huguley, C. M., Jr., and Bartolucci, A. A. Combination versus sequential five-drug chemotherapy in metastatic carcinoma of the breast. *Cancer Res.* 36:3911, 1976.
51. Smith, I. E., Fitzharris, B. M., McKinna, J. A., et al. Aminoglutethimide in treatment of metastatic breast carcinoma. *Lancet* 1:646, 1978.
52. Smith, J. A., III, Gamez-Araujo, J., Gallager, H. S., et al. Carcinoma of the breast. *Cancer* 39:527, 1977.
53. Tranum, B., Hoogstraten, B., Kennedy, A., et al. Adriamycin in combination for the treatment of breast cancer. *Cancer* 41:2078, 1978.

54. Valagussa, P., Bonadonna, G., and Veronesi, U. Patterns of relapse and survival following radical mastectomy. *Cancer* 41:1170, 1978.
55. Yonemoto, R. H., Tan, M. S. C., Byron, R. L., et al. Randomized sequential hormonal therapy vs. adrenalectomy for metastatic breast carcinoma. *Cancer* 39:547, 1977.

Christopher C. Gates

11. Psychological Aspects of Breast Cancer

The emotional impact of breast cancer and its treatment is enormous, bringing irreversible change to the patient and to the family unit. Some women undergo the cumulative stresses of positive biopsy, mastectomy, adjuvant chemotherapy, recurrence, possible adrenalectomy, long-term chemotherapy with alopecia and 1 to 2 days of nausea and vomiting after each treatment, subsequent recurrence, and finally widespread disease and death. Fortunately, all patients don't have all of these stresses.

This chapter reviews the literature on emotional aspects of breast cancer and then outlines a point of view that has evolved in working with breast cancer patients and their families at all stages of the disease. A mechanism of emotional action that patients and their families follow under the stress of cancer and its treatment is proposed. The fundamental statement of the chapter is that emotional reactions follow a logical mechanism of action just as physiologic reactions do. Treatment is based upon understanding the mechanism of action, making an accurate diagnosis, intervening on the basis of understanding the process, and evaluating the result.

The majority of the chapter addresses the elements of the coping process in patients. A distinction is made throughout between content and process. Content refers to the nature of a given emotional or physical activity; for example, optimism is an emotional activity and gardening is a physical activity. Process refers to how that activity helps to promote or to upset the emotional equilibrium of the patient. The content of a patient's physical and mental activity varies greatly, but each patient is constantly engaged in the process of maintaining equilibrium. This follows the laws of homeostasis as in other body systems and can be assessed and intervened upon.

This chapter is based on work supported by the Department of Surgery and the Division of Psychiatry, Brigham and Women's Hospital, and partially supported by the National Cancer Institute Contract No. 1-CN-65311 and Grant No. CA-19681.

255

Breast cancer is a chronic illness, the onset of which is treated acutely both medically and psychologically. Consequently the medical literature on the psychological aspects of breast cancer has addressed primarily the early disease course. The recent literature tends to group all terminal cancers into one psychological phenomenon and intimates a clinical consensus that, in late stage cancer, psychological responses are not strongly influenced by the site of the original lesion. This consensus is probably correct, but, on the other hand, there is a paucity of literature that addresses the intermediary phases of breast cancer, such as adjustment to home life, marital and sexual adjustment, psychological aspects of the "free period," and reactions to recurrence, hormone therapy, and chemotherapy.

Studies of delay behavior in breast cancer patients have been instituted in the hope of outlining a personality profile of women who are most likely to procrastinate in seeking medical advice after discovery of a mass [8, 11, 16, 18, 19, 35]. This endeavor has proved largely unsuccessful, as delay has been related to (1) familial situation, (2) age, (3) socioeconomic status, (4) educational level, (5) sense of body image, (6) habitual denial, (7) depression, and (8) multiple psychological factors. Of interest is that four studies have indicated that delayers tend to have a greater incidence of malignancies than nondelayers [1, 8, 18, 35], raising the question of whether some women are, at some unconscious level, "aware" of the pathology of the mass.

The early literature on mastectomy consisted of observations made by investigators of small populations of patients [4–6, 21, 26, 32, 39]. They avoided specific conclusions, rather describing the broad range of psychological responses immediately postmastectomy. Shock, guilt, anger, denial, loss of feminine self-image, and occasional depression were reported as common and expected reactions that the authors urged not be interpreted as maladaptive unless they developed into chronic behavior. Severe depressive reactions have been correlated with a premorbid degree of dependency and with the inability to maintain compensatory defenses [37].

The literature has been equally unsuccessful in evaluating the impact of breast loss as a variable independent of the impact of the diagnosis of cancer. Because of the double threat of breast cancer as a body mutilation and death threat, it has been repeatedly observed that a common defense mechanism of mastectomy patients is to choose to perceive breast loss as a trade-off in the face of the greater danger: "If it means saving my life, it's worth it." Clinical observers have differed on whether breast loss is more disruptive to older [24, 39] or younger [21, 33] women. Breast loss is seen as most devastating when physical appearance has been the single most important factor in a woman's total self-image [6, 14, 36]. Indeed, there is some evidence that the impact of mastectomy is not upon body image as much as it is upon total self-concept, as discussed later in this chapter. A study using psychological testing failed to detect any change in body image preoperatively and postoperatively, although self-concept was seen to decline [30]. Too, observations of women who have undergone breast reconstruction have emphasized a restored self-assertiveness and confidence rather than any increased sense of femininity [15].

Defense mechanisms are known to play a role in reducing the stress of diagnosis and treatment of breast cancer [6, 20, 37]. Denial is cited as the most commonly used, but each patient usually uses a number of defenses. The relationship between the outside stress of breast cancer, the psychological response, the defenses used to cope with the stress response, and eventual life adjustment, however, is not addressed in depth in the literature. It is one of the focal points of this chapter.

The symbolic and physical role of the breast in sexual activity has led to a focus on the sexual adjustment of breast cancer patients [7, 12, 13, 22, 23, 29, 42]. Response to the scar post-mastectomy, by both the patient and her husband, is acknowledged as an important factor toward the return to sexual activity [13]. Failure to view the scar, first by the patient and then by the husband, is stated to lead to a reduced level of physical closeness and touching, feelings of rejection, withdrawal and counter-withdrawal, and thus a permanent loss in the sexual relationship [17]. A recent study of patients with advanced cancer demonstrated that although desire for sexual intercourse decreased subsequent to diagnosis, the desire for nonsexual physical closeness increased [25], underscoring the importance to cancer patients of maintaining a physical relationship with their partners. The impact of breast cancer on husbands is a particularly neglected area, although the concerns of the breast cancer patient's spouse can be many [27].

The social adjustment of the breast cancer patient is another area of interest, and investigators usually refer to the long-term impact of the disease as the "quality of survival." The conclusions made from these investigations largely depend on the variables chosen to measure social adjustment in terms of mood, work, social and leisure activities, interpersonal relationships, and so on. The concept of measures of psychosocial outcome in breast cancer has received some attention [3], and the field of instrument design for the psychosocial assessment of oncology patients has been led by Derogatis [10]. However, the difficulties in this field are many, including the broad age range of the population, the strong intervening variables of disease course and treatment modality, and the ambiguity of the concept of "quality of life" itself.

The work that has been conducted thus far provides some evidence that mood disturbance postmastectomy peaks at 8 weeks [40], and that maladjustment at 6 months correlates with concurrent life stresses [38]. There is evidence that emotional distress and time of return to work are related to the type of mastectomy performed; the radical mastectomy brings greater adjustment difficulties than lesser operations [41]. Follow-up studies at 5 years postmastectomy have also been conducted by mailed self-report questionnaires, with return to work as the determinant variable. It is stated that over 80 percent of mastectomy patients are able to return to work and perform daily activities [9, 34]. However, it must be kept in mind that these populations have consisted of patients with operable disease at diagnosis and who have survived for 5 years. This represents only about 40 percent of the total number of breast cancer patients [2]. Little attention has been paid to the quality of life of breast cancer patients undergoing more intensive treatment for more extensive disease [28, 31]. Although the eventual survival of these patients is lower, it does not mean that efforts should not be directed toward maintaining the quality of their lives throughout the course of their illness.

In summary, the literature to date, including the observations made in this chapter, are largely descriptive and anecdotal, with various suggestions for the improved psychological management of the breast cancer patient. The current trend in management is toward more systematic assessment of psychological variables, the establishment of measures of psychosocial outcome for comparison of various management approaches, and

the eventual identification of patients at high risk for maladjustment subsequent to breast cancer diagnosis. Once the assessment of psychosocial variables has been demonstrated to
be reliable in an oncology population, hypotheses put forth in
the observational literature can be tested by more rigorous sci-
entific methods.

The Patient

The average age for occurrence of breast cancer is 52, but it
can occur at almost any age. Thus, it attacks a very broad age
spectrum as well as all strata of society. Much has been written
about people who have difficulty expressing hostility being "can-
cer-prone." This has not been demonstrated conclusively so far,
so it's wise to consider that women of all personality types are
susceptible to the disease.

Given the great variety of personality types in the general
population, the broad range of age and socioeconomic status,
and the broad spectrum of disease from stage I through stage
IV, it is not surprising that most reports on emotional aspects
of the illness stress the individuality of response and the broad
range of reactions. I have noted certain general characteristics
that seem to be common to all breast cancer patients and their
families. Keeping these in mind, it becomes possible to find
some common denominators of response and to see a logic in
the reactions of patients and their families.

As has been discussed in the literature, the illness and treatment are emotional stresses that are cumulative. It is generally
considered that about 1 in 5 of the normal adult population has
some mental illness. This means that up to 20 percent of those
who develop breast cancer will have a predisposition to difficulty
in handling emotional distress and can be expected to have more
difficulty than most in handling the emotional impact of breast
cancer and its treatment. One way to characterize mental illness
is as an increased difficulty in handling the stress of daily life.
Anyone, for that matter, who has lived with a preexisting chronic
stress (e.g., diabetes, arthritis, congenital deformity) or demonstrated difficulty handling inner distress (previous depression)
can be considered at risk for having difficulty in adjusting to
their illness and treatment.

The emotional distress one notes in cancer patients, secondary to the stress of illness and treatment, can be considered a form of inner outrage. In a sense this is self-evident. It is outrageous for anyone to develop and have to live with breast cancer. This outrage can be considered a form of inner energy, which is manifested by mental and physical activities that can either be helpful or destructive to the patient. One of the patient's tasks is to harness this increased reservoir of inner energy. The patient's outrage can be nurtured by her renewed realization that life is short and that she desires to achieve certain goals during her lifetime. Every physician is aware of instances in which patients faced with terrible misfortune and a shortened life expectancy become strongly motivated in their accomplishments. A person is faced with a life crisis that can serve as a focal point of either emotional growth or deterioration. This is the point at which the adaptive or maladaptive response arises. *Coping* is the term that will be used to describe this harnessing of activity. People who cope well are able to handle their more negative feelings in a way that is not harmful to themselves or others and can compensate for their losses in ways that are beneficial.

Mental Coping: Unconsciously Motivated

Coping includes both mental and physical activities that are either unconsciously or consciously motivated. Emotional defenses are the unconscious mental processes, while attitudes and beliefs are the conscious mental processes. Emotional defenses are an everyday coping maneuver and a prominent part of the mental status of the breast cancer patient. They are defined as mechanisms of adaptation selected unconsciously, operated automatically, to manage anxiety, aggressive impulses, hostilities, resentments, frustrations. Although everyone uses defenses, a specific defensive style gives some indication of how successfully people will cope with their illness and treatment. *Denial,* for instance, is an essential mechanism if one is to live with cancer. If a patient were in constant emotional contact with the full, grim reality of having a life-threatening illness, disfiguring treatment, and the hostile, resentful feelings that these losses produce, daily living would be very difficult. The patient would be so preoccupied with these realities that other thoughts and feelings of living would become less available. Denial is not present or absent in each patient, but it can fade in or out, depending on the need to reduce emotional stress. In fact, the patient who is adapting well is able to utilize denial in a flexible manner, to gradually accept reality at times when she feels sufficiently strong to deal with it.

Another distinction has not been made in the literature in the discussion of denial. Denial can take two forms: (1) the denial of reality: "I had cancer, but they got it all and I'm fine now" and (2) the denial of affect: "Yes, I have cancer, but what can you do about it? I don't let it bother me." The former takes on the characteristics of psychosis and is generally reflective of greater distress than the latter, in which denial is being used as an effective coping mechanism. This latter type of denial is healthy to the degree that it blots out the details and sting of the reality without sacrificing other normal functioning and without jeopardizing health. As long as the patient seeks adequate treatment for her illness, works hard to maintain as normal and balanced a life as possible, it does not matter if she is not constantly aware of her illness, scars, and uncertain future. However, if the patient has delayed in seeking medical assistance, either at the appearance of the initial lesion or at the hint of recurrence, an unhealthy denial may have played a role.

The defensive system is one that is subject to only minor changes through even intense psychological intervention. There is little room in the normal treatment of breast cancer for patients to enter into psychotherapy to attempt a restructuring of defensive functioning. As a general rule, if a patient has used denial in a maladaptive way previously to handle stress, it will take active and persistent intervention on the physician's part to get her to have frequent check-ups, and he must give careful instruction to report any new symptoms in order to prevent denial jeopardizing her care.

The person who is prone to blame others for her own failings or distress, or who imagines that her serious condition is harder for others than for herself, is employing the defense of *projection*. As with denial, a modicum of projection is reasonably healthy. Projection usually can be identified by the nurses when the patient is in the hospital. Such women are the chronic complainers who find fault with the nursing, the food, the hospital, noise, and so on. This type of behavior can therefore usually be detected on the medical chart when the nurse has indicated an excessive number of complaints on the part of the patient. Such people generally are preoccupied with feelings of inadequacy and unsatisfactory qualities in themselves, which is aggravated by the diagnosis of cancer and the treatment involved. They then project these feelings of inadequacy onto the environment. A projecter easily gets others quite angry and, if married, can be quite difficult for her spouse and family to handle.

In such cases particularly, husbands benefit from some instruction on their wives' way of handling hostility, and they can be instructed to resist being "too nice" and to set some limits on their wives when they become difficult. It seems that often such women are married to reasonably passive men who in some ways welcome being picked on. They feel that it is their role to absorb this hostility since they are not sick and they "can take it." Such interactions are reasonably difficult to change with treatment since it's a lifestyle. The problem is, however, that the "nice" husband thus encourages his wife's hostile projections to meet his own need, and the patient then feels guilty on some level for being so negative and difficult. Individuals close to the patient can be taught to set limits and to risk incurring the patient's hostility by saying "no" or "stop, I won't allow that abuse," and so on, therefore bringing under control hostile forces that the patient cannot fully manage herself. The woman who projects often has a scapegoat. Such a target person is frequently a man who is best identified when the intensity of the hostility toward him is greater than one would expect from the facts. The hostility may also be directed to a political issue or cause, when the patient suddenly becomes strongly incensed about a worldly injustice or inequality. Although this kind of projection can be constructive, it can also be seen to reflect the patient's expression of anger at the misfortune that has been dealt to her personally.

Projection also is involved in situations in which patients don't want certain family members to be told the facts, or family members don't want the patient to know the facts of the illness. It is fairly clear that the protected person usually knows just what the facts are. It often happens that the people who are seeking the protection of secrecy for someone else are actually looking to protect themselves. Some of these situations can be quite difficult to manage; they can put the physician in a difficult position when the patient or family demand that the physician hold a confidence and thus not be truthful to the other party.

Distortion, another fundamental defense, can also be troublesome to patients. In the first few days postmastectomy, no one is too troubled when some patients report relief that the tumor is not malignant when clearly they have been told otherwise. In some patients, however, distortion continues and results in major misunderstandings about diagnosis and treatment plans. When a patient has demonstrated this tendency, the observant physician notes this and takes special pains to clarify diagnostic and treatment issues with the patient and relatives to prevent, or at least to minimize, misunderstanding. However, almost every physician has dealt with the resistant case, the patient who interprets what is said to her according to her preconceived notion. In such situations, the physician is sometimes better off if he realizes that the patient needs to hold on to the distortion to maintain her own equilibrium. When such a conclusion is reached, it may be wise to secure witnesses when obtaining consent to medical procedures in order to avoid litigation, for although the patient may at the time seem to have a clear understanding of what was stated, she may later testify strongly that she heard something else altogether. The patient is not lying, for she firmly believes her statements to be true, but the use of distortion as a defense mechanism can be entirely motivated on the unconscious level.

Distortion is also a particularly troublesome defense when, in using it, patients seek the advice of several physicians for the treatment of their illness. On the one hand, it's to be recognized that doctors differ in their own judgments of the optimal treatment of breast cancer and that there is a continuing controversy over local excision and radiation versus mastectomy. In addition, doctors themselves sometimes use distortion without realizing it. Given these variables, however, it's important to be aware of possible patient distortion when reporting one physician's recommendation to another physician. Distortion should be suspected when the patient reports back that different doctors have different points of view and she does not know what course to follow. This presents a particularly hard problem for the physician because of the number of variables involved and the difficulty in obtaining all the facts. Physicians generally solve these difficulties in intuitive and common sense ways for themselves. There is little value in confronting the patient with it since this will simply raise hostility and generally serve no useful end. Once the process has been "diagnosed," however, it's important to keep it in mind when stresses occur. The prudent physician tempers his interpretation of the patient's report with this in mind.

We have described three fundamental defenses—denial, projection, and distortion—that patients fall back on at times of acute stress when their systems are in danger of being overwhelmed. Use of these defenses is then increased, and flexible defenses are decreased. When reality is significantly compromised, the patient is considered to be psychotic. It is well to remember, however, the whimsical distinction between neurosis and psychosis. "Neurosis occurs in those of us who build our castles in the sky; psychosis is in those of us who live there." The point is that the homeostatic force that allows one to be able to live comfortably with oneself is the predominant drive that prevails. A psychotic reaction in the breast cancer patient is simply a safe withdrawal to that castle in the sky that is a safer, more comfortable emotional domicile than the place in which she is faced with the unacceptable realities of disease and pain in one's body and emotional stresses in one's life.

Such a reaction occurred in a 28-year-old married woman postmastectomy. She had had one stillbirth child after her surgery and had a second pregnancy terminated when she developed metastases and underwent adrenalectomy. Her marriage, occurring after she developed breast cancer, had not been a happy one. Subsequent to (1) being told that she was not a candidate for pregnancy, (2) recurrence of her disease, and (3) treatment with chemotherapy and subsequent hair loss, she developed the delusion that her family could no longer care for her since she was such a burden. She was quite sure that a bombing reported in the local newspapers occurred as a direct result of her illness, and she was also convinced that her family and her caretaking physicians were in mortal danger from imminent disaster. She required psychiatric hospitalization to manage this global distortion and projected outrage.

A second case involved a 52-year-old woman who had undergone bilateral mastectomies 12 and 13 years previously and adrenalectomy 3 years previously. Under the multiple stresses of recurrent disease; the sixteenth birthday of her youngest son, a symbolic loss of his dependency; the anniversary of her mother's death from breast cancer; and loss of her best friend from breast cancer, the patient developed a delusion that her husband was having an affair. While the situation was difficult for her husband, the delusion allowed her to project venomous outrage upon him and in some ways allowed her to handle the enormous inner distress that was being generated.

These are the unusual cases, however, and in most patients denial, projection, and distortion do not reach psychotic levels. The more flexible defenses of rationalization, displacement, reaction-formation, disassociation of affect, and sublimation are also evident when the stress is being managed capably. These are considered the "neurotic" defenses that are used to manage anxiety. Examples are (1) reaction-formation: "I've heard of women who get really angry at their surgeons, but I could never get mad at Dr. ———; he's so nice; I really love him." (2) isolation of affect: "Of course, everyone who gets cancer is sure they're going to die, and mastectomy can be a real blow to a woman, but what can you do?" (3) suppression: "I don't like to think about it; I don't let myself think about it." (4) rationalization: "Every time I feel sorry for myself, I remember all those people I saw down in radiation therapy." (5) sublimation: "I was mad, but I saw that wasn't going to get me anywhere. Our family has really been brought closer since my operation; we don't bicker about the small things like we used to." (6) intellectualization: "The statistics are in my favor so I shouldn't have to worry so much."

In patients in whom defenses are noted to change drastically, it is usually from the more flexible defenses of rationalization, intellectualization, and so on, toward the more rigid and potentially psychotic defenses of denial, projection, and distortion. In such instances the physican should look for a concurrent life crisis or cumulative stress that has added to the stress of breast cancer and forced a more rigid coping response. This process usually passes with the abatement of the concurrent crisis and should not be interpreted as a permanent change in coping behavior. However, the large disruption in family life that such strong defenses can produce often requires immediate intervention.

Overwhelming distress can lead to a total defensive breakdown. At this point, previously unacknowledged feelings can become manifest, often severe depression or acute anger. As with defensive change, times of defensive failure are also usually temporary. By admitting to previously unexpressed feelings, the patient is able to get some insight and now has the opportunity to act upon those feelings. Defensive functioning is usually restored after a while. However, as was stated in the discussion of the literature review, the failure to maintain compensatory defenses has been correlated with maladjustment postmastectomy. It is thus possible that defenses serve to buffer the patient from depression as well as alleviate stress. Defenses are thus considered to be fundamental emotional balancing mechanisms that help patients and family members cope with their inner distress in ways in which they can most successfully maintain a sense of emotional balance and equilibrium.

Defenses are inherent in all personality styles and are used to cope with everyday life stresses. However, with a diagnosis of breast cancer and the stress that that diagnosis brings, the operation of defenses becomes apparent on a level manifest to the trained observer. Although alteration of defensive styles is not possible in a medical setting, the identification and monitoring of specific defenses can assist the physician in patient management. For example, the physician can postpone certain stressful courses of treatment if it is clear that the patient is already experiencing considerable distress and is using considerable denial or distortion. He may also help family members not to allow excessive projection or distortion on the part of the patient to disrupt their daily life and can give them permission to set limits on the patient when necessary.

As has been stated, psychotic maneuvers are also a way of communicating distress and can therefore be interpreted as a plea for emotional support. As with other homeostatic processes (ecologic or physiologic) the defenses are part of an emotional system that can handle marginal levels of stress. A breaking down or a going out of control of defensive function, however, is indicative of a breakdown of the total system; outside intervention is now required. The interrelationship between defensive functioning and the endocrinologic system has been well demonstrated by Katz and co-workers [20].

Physical Coping: Unconsciously Motivated

A component of physical activity is also unconsciously motivated and plays a role in adaptation. This too is so close to
common sense and everyday life that seeing people's activities
as particular mechanisms might seem overly mechanistic. The
fact is, however, that once the idea of the organism striving to
maintain homeostasis is accepted and the role of activity understood, then it becomes possible to look at each person's physical
activity as well as mental activity and see it as part of a homeostatic process. It then becomes a diagnostic task to assess
whether or not optimal homeostasis is being achieved.

The relationship between stress and activity is not a new one,
and it is identified by the cliche, "When the going gets tough,
the tough get going." This is noticeable in patients, particularly
postmastectomy patients, who are determined to keep up their
physical appearance, who find themselves talking more to friends
and to relations, and who are working harder at their jobs without consciously deciding to increase their activity. It's a type of
preprogrammed response in people, in this case in those with
strong coping abilities, and it has an obvious useful result.

There are also maladaptive behaviors that people automatically employ when they are under stress. For some, it is an
emotional distancing, the result of which is cutting down contact
with other people. It's not infrequent for leisure time activity
to lose appeal and to decline. Sexual interest also often dimin-
ishes, and patients find themselves not returning to whatever
was their level of previous sexual contact. If patients or spouses
had a tendency to abuse themselves with alcohol or drugs in
times of distress, these behaviors or habits often recur. As a
general rule, those forces in patients and spouses that in the
past may have tended to work against them when they were
under stress and were dealing with inner distress, will do so
again, and will become more intense as the stresses and inner
distress increase.

Mental and Physical Coping: Consciously Motivated

It is in the consciously motivated mental and physical activities
that the physician and other caretakers have the greatest input.
It is here that instruction, example, encouragement, support,

and so on can become a very useful part of the everyday care-taking practice of physicians.

Beliefs and attitudes are considered conscious mental coping mechanisms. Maintaining hope of a realistic, desired outcome is considered an essential ingredient in maintaining emotional equilibrium and combatting depressive feelings. An optimistic or hopeful view can be maintained and can shift as circumstances shift. This ability to shift is a key ingredient and one in which the psychiatric term *ego strength* is very much involved. Those patients adapt the best who can shift responses as the reality changes. Even though the content of the hope may differ, the process continues. As an example, someone with this capacity can hope that the lump when first discovered is benign. If it is benign, the hope is fulfilled; if it's malignant, however, then they can hope that the nodes aren't involved. This "shifting of gears" can be continued throughout the course of disease. If necessary, the last hope is that pain will not be great, that perhaps one's belief in an afterlife will be true, that one's family will be able to manage, and so on. What is important is not the particular content of the hope, but the capacity to generate hope, to be able to shift as circumstances shift, and to maintain that positive feeling.

Other conscious coping activities are those that restore injured body image or self-esteem. There are many opportunities available to a woman who has had a mastectomy to maintain her physical appearance. She can investigate types of prostheses to find the one most suitable for her individual figure. She can adapt her wardrobe to her prosthesis or she can look into the possibility of reconstructive surgery. The enthusiastic interest in mastectomy fashion shows illustrates the need for this sort of information. If the patient feels that there is no way she can feel as sexy or attractive as she did before her mastectomy, she may compensate for this loss by investing more intense efforts into a career or interpersonal life. As stated earlier, the energy made available from the inner outrage at her adversity can motivate her to greater accomplishments than she had previously strived for.

These observations may seem so basic as to be almost trite, but maintaining physical appearance and undertaking compensating activities are important parts of the coping process. In observing the interchange between the personnel in surgeons' offices and their breast cancer patients, it was clear that emotional support was intuitively provided by a comment on a new wig, a compliment on a few lost pounds, or an inquiry about the patient's favorite hobby. It is worthwhile to find out those activities and relationships that contribute most to a patient's self-esteem and that she most enjoys. By monitoring these sources of self-esteem at each follow-up visit, physicians can quickly pick up on adjustment difficulties. Clearly, the woman who gained enormous satisfaction from her garden prior to her illness but who states that she just hasn't gotten around to it this year is indicating that she is not adapting well.

Although the instinctual drive to maintain a favorable self-concept motivates most women to pursue self-gratifying activities, the injury of breast cancer occasionally initiates a chain of self-destructive events that drain self-esteem completely. This is what has occurred in the woman who withdraws from relationships that have been important to her, who gives up any attempt to look good in public, who sees no purpose in continuing on her job, and who loses all faith in God or the future. This is the "hopeless and helpless" patient who develops into a burden on family and physicians, although such a reaction is not restricted to patients with breast cancer. Physicians may be tempted to let such patients leave the medical system because of the effort required to change this kind of attitude. It is sometimes helpful in these cases to have the social worker set up a family conference and instruct the family to make the patient accountable for her own behavior. The "victimized" patient will continue in her rampage as long as those around her reinforce the attitude that she is being victimized.

Terminal Stages

As has been said earlier, later stage breast cancer patients are not specifically different from any cancer patient in the end stages of the disease. The disease has spread, often to bone with the possibility of considerable pain. Chemotherapy and radiation have been used with variable success, and eventually the disease in many patients has progressed to end stage. Imminent death is the ultimate stress to one's sense of self. Dying with dignity, dying gracefully, and so on are considered here as dying with optimal coping strategies operating. I believe that there is no right or proper way to die, as such. Dying is an individual process of coping, just as is living.

People generally die in the same patterns as they have lived. The gregarious and outgoing person is more likely to have friends and relatives around her at death than the generally isolated, more solitary person. The person who is able to express feelings and is in touch with a broad range of emotional responses in her lifetime will be more likely to be able to talk about her fears of dying, fears of the unknown, and so on. It is unreasonable to expect that the person who has a defensive configuration such that these feelings of anxiety were not available to them for discussion when they were not ill will have them available when death is anticipated.

Patients pass through stages of dying, to some extent, in the familiar sequence of denial, anger, bargaining, acceptance, and so on, described by Kübler-Ross. These are considered a sequence of coping strategies involving primarily defensive functioning with attitudes and beliefs often playing an important role. In the end, though, it is usually the early, conditioned attitudes and beliefs that come to the fore. An example is a woman who had had a strong Catholic upbringing, but who had not been a practicing believer in her adult years. She had found meaning in transcendental meditation (TM) during the later stages of her illness. As she became terminal, however, the TM beliefs diminished and her cross and rosary appeared. Even though she had disparaged her beliefs previously, with adequate stress this belief and behavior returned as her primary coping style.

Very often patients greatly increase denial, distortion, and projection to protect themselves from frightening feelings of annihilation. At some point, these mechanisms often break down and for a period of time outrage is present. This breakdown of defenses is considered equivalent to Kübler-Ross's stage of anger. Patients who maintain successful coping strategies are more often able to mobilize compensating interpersonal, achievement, and identification activities, which can assume great importance around the time of death. This is particularly true for religious beliefs which provide a sense of purpose, meaning, continuity, and feeling cared about. These are compensating feelings about self, just when body-self is painful and deteriorating and when achievement-self usually is inactive.

The Family and Others

The impact of breast cancer is felt by those who are close to the patient as well as by the patient herself. Probably the most important ones to be affected are the spouse, if the patient is married, and those with whom she lives, if she isn't living alone. It is now recognized that a patient who lives alone does not survive as long as those who live with someone else. This is not only true for patients with breast cancer in particular, but for cancer patients in general.

The stress on a spouse is obvious. He is threatened with possible loss of his wife from cancer from the time of first diagnosis. It is expensive to have cancer and be treated for it; while most husbands naturally will gladly incur the expense if it will benefit their wives, even in cases of early cancer when most insurance policies cover hospital expenses, there is the expense of the prosthesis, clothing, and so on. Later stage cancer brings enormous cost, with doctors' bills (often not completely covered by insurance), medicine, transportation into the doctor's office and hospital, treatments, and caretakers for the home on a part-time or full-time basis. If the patient was employed and she cannot return to work, there is an added temporary or permanent loss of income. For a self-employed woman who does not have a family to support her, curtailment or loss of job over time can necessitate a complete lifestyle change and can bring on the stress of serious financial hardship in addition to the enormous stress of the illness and treatment.

These major stresses stir up feelings in the spouse that he has to deal with on some level. Very often husbands have to deal with feelings of strong resentment, and they sometimes are put in a very difficult position. There is a tendency among many caring husbands to deny their negative feelings, or to ignore them if they are aware of them, if these feelings are directed toward their wives. They tend to adopt a positive attitude, taking one day at a time and pursuing a determined posture that everything is going to be all right and that nothing has changed. This is particularly true where the wives have stage I and II cancers; at this point metastatic disease has not been diagnosed and it's much easier to figuratively blot out the whole experience. This is an adaptive coping effect, but it can have an emotional price tag for the patient. She well knows that everything isn't the same, that her mortality is threatened, and that a positive attitude from her spouse does not acknowledge this change and thus does not acknowledge her attitude. Physicians must assist husbands to understand their own hostilities and to give them permission to be angry at their wives at appropriate times, both for the benefit of the husbands as well as the wives. It is a difficult rehabilitation task to ask husbands to understand that this airing of feelings is necessary.

Another situation frequently encountered after mastectomy is a couple's difficulty in returning to their previous level of sexual functioning. What can happen is that after the couple begins foreplay, the patient will become very angry, but neither she nor her husband will understand why. What has been found in a number of such cases, after the wife's hostility has been carefully investigated, is that the wife does not believe her partner when he reports that he finds her sexually desirable and stimulating. The source of this disbelief is her own negative self-image after her mastectomy. After rejecting his viewpoint—that he does find her desirable—she then imagines that he is approaching her just to satisfy his own sexual needs and with no desire specifically for her. This then confirms her own self-devaluing feelings and suspicions and gives her permission, on an inner level, to be angry and sometimes openly furious with her husband for abusing her and using her simply for an available outlet of his sexual feelings.

For the husband, the hostility is puzzling. He often feels that if he continues to pressure her for sex, her hostility toward him will be aggravated and will lead to a further blow-up. If he chooses to leave her alone, sacrificing his own desires, then he puts himself in the position of confirming the very feelings that she imagined him to have. He is now in a seemingly impossible position. In such cases, the wife's feelings deserve to be investigated, and if it turns out that indeed she does not feel desirable and does feel abused, then these feelings should be shared with her husband. On the one hand, it's important for the husband not to press his wife, but at the same time it's not to her benefit or to his for him to give up sexual contact and not deal with the hostility.

Only through a gentle, but often-repeated, approach on his part will he convince her that it is her desire as well as his that is fostering his interest. In the process he is achieving much more than a return to sexual function. He is making a very specific self-esteem intervention for the patient that she is not able to do for herself. Particularly with mastectomy, it is clear that a woman's sexual function is a very important indicator not only for return to function but as a general guide to how well the patient is feeling about herself and how able she is to enter into close physical and emotional activity with those she loves.

Breast cancer and its treatment are emotional stresses on patients and family; these stresses are cumulative and are dealt with by a complex individual process of coping. Every woman is an individual, and the way she copes with disease and treatment are unique to her. At the same time she is also struggling to maintain emotional equilibrium, just as are other women.

Her individuality is content, the struggle for equilibrium is process. The content and process of unconsciously and consciously motivated mental and physical activity are the elements of coping. Coping style is seen as what determines one's quality of life while living with and being treated for breast cancer. It also determines the manner in which one will deal with death when it comes. This process of coping is considered to follow the same general laws of homeostasis as the other body systems. As it is understood, diagnosis and treatment of pathologic or maladaptive response can follow the same principles as used with any of the other body systems.

References

1. Aitken-Swan, J., and Peterson, R. The cancer patient: Delay in seeking advice. *Br. Med. J.* 1:623, 1955.
2. American Cancer Society. *Cancer Facts and Figures.* New York: American Cancer Society, 1976.
3. Avery, A. D., et al. *The Quality of Medical Care Assessment Using Outcome Measures: Eight Disease-Specific Applications.* Santa Monica, Calif.: Rand Corporation, 1976.
4. Bard, M. The sequence of emotional reactions in radical mastectomy patients. *Public Health Rep.* 67:1144, 1952.
5. Bard, M. The relationship of the personality factors of dependence to psychological invalidism in women following radical mastectomy. New York University, Ph.D. Thesis, 1953.
6. Bard, M., and Sutherland, A. Psychological impact of cancer and its treatment: IV. Adaptation to radical mastectomy. *Cancer* 8:656, 1955.
7. Byrd, B. F. Sex after mastectomy. *Med. Aspects Hum. Sexuality* 9:53, 1975.

8. Cameron, A., and Hinton, J. Delay in seeking treatment for mammary tumors. *Cancer* 21:1121, 1968.
9. Craig, T. J., et al. The quality of survival in breast cancer: A case-control comparison. *Cancer* 33:1451, 1974.
10. Derogatis, L. R. *PAIS: Psychosocial Adjustment to Illness Scale.* Baltimore: Clinical Psychometric Research, 1975.
11. Eardley, A. Triggers to action. A study of what makes women seek advice for breast conditions. *Int. J. Health Educ.* 17:256, 1974.
12. Ervin, C. V., Jr. Sex life after breast removal. *Sexology* 35:391, 1969.
13. Ervin, C. V., Jr. Psychological adjustment to mastectomy. *Med. Aspects Hum. Sexuality* 7:42, 1973.
14. Friel, P. B., et al. Adverse emotional reactions to disfigurative surgery: Detection and management. *Conn. Med.* 31:277, 1972.
15. Gifford, S. Emotional Attitudes Toward Cosmetic Breast Surgery: Loss and Restitution of the Ideal Self. In R. M. Goldwyn (ed.), *Plastic and Reconstructive Surgery of the Breast.* Boston: Little, Brown, 1976.
16. Gold, M. A. Causes of patients' delay in diseases of the breast. *Cancer* 17:564, 1964.
17. Grandstaff, N. W. The Impact of Breast Cancer on the Family. In J. M. Vaeth (ed.), *Breast Cancer: Its Impact on the Patient, Family and Community. Frontiers of Radiation Therapy Oncology,* Vol. 11. Basel, Switzerland: S. Karger, 1976.
18. Greer, S. Psychological aspects: Delay in the treatment of breast cancer. *Proc. R. Soc. Med.* 67:470, 1974.
19. Hammerschlag, C. A., et al. Breast symptoms and patient delay: Psychological variables involved. *Cancer* 17:1480, 1964.
20. Katz, J. L., et al. Stress, distress and ego defenses. *Arch. Gen. Psychiatr.* 23:131, 1970.
21. Kenneker, R., and Cutler, M. Psychological problems of adjustment to cancer of the breast. *J.A.M.A.* 148:833, 1952.
22. Kent, S. Coping with sexual identity crisis after mastectomy. *Geriatrics* 30:145, 1975.
23. Klein, R. A crisis to grow on. *Cancer* 28:1160, 1971.
24. Kushner, R. *Breast Cancer. A Personal History and an Investigative Report.* New York: Harcourt Brace Jovanovich, 1975.
25. Leiber, L., et al. The communication of affection between cancer patients and their spouses. *Psychosom. Med.* 38:379, 1976.
26. Lewison, E. F. The Psychological Aspects of Breast Cancer. In E. F. Lewison (ed.), *Breast Cancer and Its Diagnosis and Treatment.* New York: Williams & Wilkins, 1955.
27. Lobsenz, N. M. What will our marriage be like now? *McCall's,* August, 1973.
28. McCorkle, M. R. Coping with physical symptoms in metastatic breast cancer. *Am. J. Nurs.* 73:1034, 1973.

29. Notman, M. Psychosexual Consequences of Mastectomy. Presented at the 10th Anniversary Meeting of the Greater Baltimore Medical Center, Johns Hopkins, Sept. 1975. Unpublished data.
30. Polivy, J. Effects of radical mastectomy on a woman's feminine self-concept. Northwestern University, Master's Thesis, 1973.
31. Priestman, T. J., and Baum, M. Evaluation of quality of life in patients receiving treatment for advanced breast cancer. *Lancet* 1:899, 1976.
32. Quint, J. C. The impact of mastectomy. *Am. J. Nurs.* 63:88, 1963.
33. Schmid, M. L., et al. The team approach to rehabilitation after mastectomy. *J. Assoc. OR Nurses* 19:821, 1974.
34. Schottenfeld, D., and Robbins, G. Quality of survival among patients who have had radical mastectomy. *Cancer* 26:650, 1970.
35. Sugar, M., and Watkins, C. Some observations about patients with a breast mass. *Cancer* 14:979, 1961.
36. Sutherland, A. M. Psychological observations in cancer patients. *Int. Psychiatry Clin.* 4:75, 1967.
37. Sutherland, A. M., and Orbach, C. E. Depressive Reactions Associated with Surgery for Cancer. In *The Psychological Impact of Cancer.* (American Cancer Society Professional Education Publication.) New York: American Cancer Society, 1974.
38. Topitzer, G. The effect of psychosocial factors on the rehabilitation of the cancer patient. Columbia University Ph.D. Thesis, 1975.
39. Watkins, C. The emotional response to tumors of the breast. *J.S. Carolina Med. Assn.* 56:43, 1960.
40. Weisman, A. D., et al. The existential plight in cancer: Significance of the first 100 days. *Int. J. Psychiatry Med.* 7:1, 1977.
41. Winick, L., and Robbins, G. F. Physical and psychological readjustment after mastectomy: An evaluation of Memorial Hospital's PMRG program. *Cancer* 39:478, 1977.
42. Witkin, M. H. Sex therapy and mastectomy. *J. Sex Marital Ther.* 1:290, 1975.

Index